THAI SEX TALK
THE LANGUAGE OF SEX AND SEXUALITY IN THAILAND

T0350095

THAI SEX TALK

THE LANGUAGE OF SEX AND SEXUALITY IN THAILAND

Pimpawun Boonmongkon and Peter A. Jackson

Editors

Timo Ojanen

Translator

MEKONG PRESS

Mekong Press was initiated in 2005 by Silkworm Books with the financial support of the Rockefeller Foundation. In 2007, the Mekong Press Foundation was registered as a nonprofit organization to encourage and support the work of local scholars, writers, and publishing professionals in Cambodia, Laos, Vietnam, and the other countries in the Greater Mekong Subregion. Books published by Mekong Press (www.mekongpress.com) are marketed and distributed internationally. Mekong Press also holds seminars and training workshops on different aspects of book publishing, and helps find ways to overcome some of the huge challenges faced by small book publishers in the region.

The publication of this book was funded by the Rockefeller Foundation.

ISBN: 978-616-90053-5-3

Published in 2012 by
Mekong Press
6 Sukkasem Road, T. Suthep
Chiang Mai 50200 Thailand
info@mekongpress.com
http://www.mekongpress.com

Cover design by Lisa Carta

Typeset in Minion Pro 10.5 pt. by Silk Type
Printed and bound in China

5 4 3 2 1

CONTENTS

CONTENTS

PREFACE

I am neither an academic nor a researcher, just a writer with an interest in sexual matters. I'm preoccupied by them: lust, vice, and craving—three sins the Lord Buddha often spoke about. Reading *Thai Sex Talk: The Language of Sex and Sexuality in Thailand*, I was amazed at the depth at which the researchers have studied sexual matters, and the choice of words as the basis of the analysis.

I like words because I need them when I write, but I usually turn to literature to find them. Sometimes I don't understand them, or can't use them correctly. Some words are "private" not "public" and, as a journalist, I can't use such words. Researchers, on the other hand, can use private words without having to be afraid of a reaction from the public. I'd like Thai people to be able to use all the words in the Thai language, whether in writing or in speech, in public or in private, especially words that relate to gender, sexuality, and health. Because figurative language is common in Thai, there is no need to always use words with literal meanings. This use of figurative language is one of the charms of the Thai language. It beautifully reduces obscenity, while allowing accurate communication.

This study of sexual language in Thai society is highly commendable and should be disseminated to the public as widely as possible, since Thai society is still in the dark about sexual matters and so many people follow double standards. If other studies are similarly published, they will collectively serve Thai society as a manual for the correct use of language in communicating about sexual matters. Then, these matters will be handled more openly and in a more informed manner.

When we know sexual terminology more broadly and deeply, we will have a new perspective for talking and writing, and Thai society will finally realize that sexual matters are not private, mysterious, or disgraceful. I think that this book is important because it will help one become more tolerant and accommodating of those with a gender or sexuality different from one's own. It can free us from prejudice and hatred, and through this promote and improve the sexual health of Thai people.

Niwat Kongphian
Columnist, *Matichon Sut Sapda*

FOREWORD

In building understanding on gender, sexuality, sexual rights, and health, problems can arise if people working on these issues lack understanding of the terms used to describe sexual practices, societal beliefs regarding sexual matters, and the power inequalities that exist in constructing the language that we use in communicating issues of gender and sexuality in our everyday lives. We sometimes perpetuate misconceptions about gender and sexuality through the use of such language without being aware of it.

The original Thai version of this book was the third Thai-language study by the Southeast Asian Consortium on Gender, Sexuality, and Health, and the first one to present the consortium's own research in book form. This study presents the research team's analyses of the sociocultural construction of gender and sexuality through the creation and use of language in the Thai context. By bringing together people and institutions in the countries of Southeast Asia and China, the consortium aims to enhance knowledge, build capacity, and promote understanding concerning gender, sexuality, and health in these countries. The consortium works in three main ways. First, it arranges short leadership training courses on gender, sexuality, and health (in two formats: fully international courses and bilingual Thai/Lao courses). Second, it trains and funds young researchers who study sexuality, gender, and health in its member countries. Third, it publishes books and other print materials that disseminate knowledge about these topics in its member countries.

The consortium's determination to work on gender, sexuality, and health through research, training, and advocacy—so as to integrate these issues into policy making as well as various projects and campaigns on rights and reproductive and sexual health—is also an important goal for the Center for Health Policy Studies, which acts as the consortium's secretariat. The consortium and the Center for Health Policy Studies have collaborated with research teams in the Philippines, Indonesia, and Vietnam to study sexuality keywords in order to increase understanding of how the use of language constructs beliefs and practices related to gender and sexuality in each country.

The research team extends its thanks to those who have helped this project succeed in its goals: Suwannee Hanmusicwatkoon, consortium coordinator for this project, and Jetsada Taesombat, consortium program assistant for the project. Two academics also helped to provide advice and gather terminology from the viewpoints of feminism and regional culture: Niporn Sanhajareya and Soiboon Saithong. Gracious thanks are also extended Dr. Michael Tan, head of the Department of Anthropology, Faculty of Sociology and Philosophy, the University of the Philippines, who persuaded the research team to participate in the Sexuality Keywords project, and to The Ford Foundation, which provided financial assistance for the research project that led to the publication of this book.

Pimpawun Boonmongkon
Founding Member
Southeast Asian Consortium on Gender, Sexuality, and Health

TRANSLATOR'S NOTES

This translation is a slightly abridged version of the original Thai text. The order of the chapters has been revised to provide a more sequenced introduction to the key features and patterns of Thai sexual culture for readers who are unfamiliar with Thai culture. Some explanatory notes have also been incorporated into the text to help clarify certain terms, ideas, and sociocultural settings. This English edition contains somewhat more detailed reference information than the Thai edition; however, in some cases it was not possible to find full reference data, which explains the incompleteness of some citations. Wherever possible, the translations provide equivalent English terms of the same register as the Thai original. That is, polite and formal Thai expressions have been rendered in formal English, and colloquial Thai expressions have been given roughly comparable English renderings.

All relevant Thai terms are introduced in romanized form in italics followed by Thai script in parentheses the first time they appear. There is no generally agreed-upon system for representing Thai in roman script, and all existing systems have some limitations. This book follows a modified version of the Royal Institute of Thailand's romanization system.[1] This system makes no distinction between long and short vowel forms, and tones are not represented. We differ from the Royal Institute system in some respects, such as using "*jor jan*" (not "*ch*") and "*eu,*" "*eua,*" "*euay*" (not "*ue,*" "*uea,*" "*ueay*") for these vowels and diphthongs. There are also certain other minor differences from the Royal Institute system. Dashes are used to separate the units of Thai compound expressions that are translated as a single term in English, such as *khwam-pen-thai* for "Thainess" and *phu-ying* for "woman." While Thai does not mark grammatical number, with no difference between singular and plural forms of nouns, we have added an English "s" to certain transcribed Thai terms that have a plural sense in order to accord with English grammatical conventions.

To avoid possible confusion and to follow commonly used romanized spellings, several words are rendered in ways that do not agree with the modified Royal Institute system used elsewhere in this translation, for example:

ดี้—*dee*, not *di*

หี—*hee*, not *hi*

อี—*ee*, not *i*

Included at the end of the book for reference is a glossary and index of Thai terms arranged in alphabetical order according to their romanized spellings.

We follow the Thai academic norm of referring to Thai authors by given names, not surnames, and all citations by Thai authors are alphabetized in the bibliography and elsewhere by given names. We also follow Thai authors' preferred spellings of their names in roman script when this is known, even if these spellings are not consistent with the modified Royal Institute system used here to transcribe other terms.

Translated entries from Thai dictionaries use n. for *noun*, v. for *verb*, adj. for *adjective*, syn. for *synonym*, coll. for *colloquial*, lit. for *literal*, met. for *metaphorical*, P. for Pali, and S. for Sanskrit.

Thai words that have been borrowed from English are italicized (e.g., *gay*, *swinging*, *tom*), and the original English spellings of these terms are preserved even if they may be pronounced somewhat differently in Thai. Borrowed words often take on distinct nuances in Thai, and this distinctiveness is signaled by placing them in italics. For example, while in English "swinging" may mean either "to be trendy and up to date" or "to engage in partner swapping," in Thai, *swinging* refers only to partner swapping.

In Thai, the terms for "man" (*phu-chai*) and "woman" (*phu-ying*) imply "heterosexual man" and "heterosexual woman," respectively. The use of the English terms "man" and "woman" in this translation should be read as denoting heterosexual preference unless otherwise specified. In Thai, *gay* is opposed to "man" (*phu-chai*) because the former denotes homosexual preference, while the latter implies heterosexual preference. The combination "gay man" (*phu-chai gay*) is a non sequitur in Thai and does not occur. We use the expression a "*gay*," rather than the standard English a "*gay* man," to avoid confusing the heterosexual nuances of the term "man" (*phu-chai*) with the homosexual preference that is denoted by the word "gay." We also follow Thai usage in using *gay* as both a noun, for male homosexual identity, and as an adjective.

Translating the key Thai term *phet* presents something of a challenge, as in different settings it may denote either "sex," "gender," or "sexuality." In some contexts *phet* may also mean both gender and sexuality. We have taken the context of usage into account in determining whether to translate *phet* as either "sex," "gender," "sexuality," or "gender and sexuality." Men who love men (*chai rak chai*), women who love women (*ying rak ying*), and the transgendered and transsexual (*phu-ying praphet sorng*) are now often referred to collectively as *khon thi mi khwam-lak-lai thang-phet*, and this expression occurs frequently in the this text. While "LGBT" (lesbian, gay, bisexual, transgender/transsexual) and "queer people" are rough English equivalents of this expression, we have chosen to preserve the sense of the Thai original and translate it as "people of diverse genders and sexualities."

The translator wishes to thank Isnai Kraisem, Phra Waradham, and the authors and editors for their kind assistance with the translation process.

Timo Ojanen

INTRODUCTION TO THE THAI EDITION

Pimpawun Boonmongkon
Project Investigator

Communication about sexual matters (*reuang phet*) is not confined to private spaces. Contrary to what is generally thought in Thailand, these matters are not taboo subjects. In fact, they are talked about in all contexts and are related to every aspect of life. Many issues that we might not think are sexual matters in one way or another are, in fact, related to them, because sexual matters do not just mean intercourse. Sexual matters, or what academics call "sexuality" (*phet-withi*), include anatomical and sex role differences, belief systems, the assigning of meanings, sexual identities, relationships, tastes, desires, and behaviors. We thus talk about them all the time, whether we are aware of it or not.

It is generally accepted that both the spoken and written language have important roles in constructing sexualities and our beliefs about them. This series of studies of power, rights, and sexual health through Thai sexuality keywords is part of a larger research project, the Southeast Asian and Chinese Sexuality Keywords Project, led by Dr. Michael Tan from the University of the Philippines. In this project, researchers from Indonesia, Vietnam, the Philippines, and Thailand have studied local languages in relation to sexual matters and sexualities. The language-use contexts studied were diverse, including language used in homes, within families, with friends, on the streets, in places of worship, on the TV and radio, on the telephone, in newspapers and magazines, as well as in academic writing, advocacy campaigns, and health services.

The term "keywords" comes from Marxist anthropologist Raymond Williams, who defined it as groups of words that are important in explaining and interpreting various phenomena and activities in order to exhibit the implicit ideas and ideologies behind them.[1] Anna Wierzbicka defines "keywords" as terms that are important and persist within a culture, but which people have little awareness of in terms of their prevalence and continual use in everyday life.[2] They can be compared to the hidden structures of thought that direct the behavior of people living in the society in question. French sociologist Pierre Bourdieu has called them "practical knowledge," that is, a mechanism that is programed by our thoughts and that unconsciously modifies our behavior.[3]

This project has involved systematic study, analysis, and awareness building with regard to various aspects of sexuality. These include:

- the sexual culture of Thailand: sexual beliefs, definitions, and practices that reflect other aspects of society and culture, e.g., gender order, social class, values, and ethnicity;
- the differences and similarities in sexual beliefs, definitions, and practices that individuals or groups have;
- cross-cultural and cross-regional comparisons; the social construction of sexual culture and sexuality, and its consequences with regard to sexual rights and sexual health, and the provision of sexual health services; and
- the power language has to change ideas, beliefs, definitions, and practices related to sexual matters.

Thai Sex Talk: The Language of Sex and Sexuality in Thailand studies everyday gender and sexuality keywords, including their history, who created them and for what purposes, their explicit and implicit meanings, for whom and in which contexts each word is used, and related terms. Analysis focuses on how these terms affect gender- and sexuality-related ideas, beliefs, definitions, and practices, as well as sexual rights, sexual and reproductive health, and the provision of health services.

Research Methodology

In choosing the keywords to be studied, three criteria were used. Each word had to be a widely used everyday term related to sexual matters, gender, or sexuality; have a meaning that is still debated within Thai society; or have been recently created to communicate a new viewpoint on sexual matters or to deconstruct misconceptions about gender and/or sexuality.

Altogether, twenty-one keywords were chosen and accompanied by related terms. The keywords fall into the following four broad categories: dominant cultural attitudes to sexuality, sexual physiology, sexual identities and roles, and sexual practices and new types of sexual relationships.

Twenty-one words may seem like a small sample to represent a sexual meaning system that interlinks with every dimension of life. Yet these terms reflect every aspect of the Thai sexual meaning system, including sexual organs (*hee, khuay*); the evaluation of bodies (*eum, po*); gender and sexual identities (*ying rak ying, chai rak chai, kathoey, sopheni*); gender and cultural values on sexual matters (*rak nuan sa-nguan tua, sin sort, kheun khan, Khun Phaen*); sexual relationships (*kik*); sexual roles, emotions, and desires (*heun, set*); various types of sexual activity (*chuay tua-eng, ao kan, chai pak, tui, swinging*); and broad umbrella concepts like *reuang phet* that defy attempts to pin down their meaning precisely.

In this study, the meaning of each keyword is first defined and the term's history is evaluated in relation to similar terms, those who have coined the terms, and the users of each term. This is followed by a deconstruction of the term's meaning, using critical theories of gender and sexuality as analytical tools. Finally, the implications of the meanings and usage of terms with regard to sexual health are considered in the context of the sexual misconceptions that are perpetuated by the patriarchal structure of Thai society and culture.

The study uses a qualitative methodology and critical feminist and queer theory for analysis and interpretation. Data collection combined three approaches:

Archival study, using data from academic materials, newspapers, websites, and web boards.

Collation of experiences from research projects, conferences, and training sessions, particularly from: (i) a project for providing reproductive health care to rural people, in a collaboration between the Center for Health Policy Studies and Nam Phong Hospital, Khon Kaen Province, between 2000 and 2005; and (ii) from a workshop on sexual pleasure, which was part of the second short Thai-Lao training course on gender, sexuality, and sexual health, arranged by the Southeast Asian Consortium on Gender, Sexuality, and Health.

Focus groups, that discussed sexuality, gender, sexual health, and/or AIDS with participants that were comprised of:

Group 1: Ten HIV/AIDS activists from Northern Thailand
Group 2: Five activists from Bangkok and Pattaya engaged in advocacy

work on the human rights of people of diverse genders and
sexualities

Group 3:   Fifty members of the Thai Women and HIV/AIDS Task Force,
consisting of people living with HIV/AIDS and of HIV/AIDS
advocates from Ubon Ratchathani Province.

The research team consisted of researchers experienced in fieldwork, facilitators
of training courses related to gender and sexuality, and activists working on
social and policy issues related to gender, sexuality, sexual rights, reproductive
health, gender-based violence against women, AIDS, and homosexuality. The
researchers' experiences and identities were diverse in a range of domains. In
terms of gender and sexual identities our researchers included heterosexual men
(*phu-chai*), heterosexual women (*phu-ying*), men who love men (*chai rak chai*),
and women who love women (*ying rak ying*). Some were single while others had a
partner, and they came from all four major geographical regions of the Thailand:
the central region, the north, the northeast (Isan), and the south. This diversity
enabled the team to engage in deep analysis that was specific yet comprehensive
and also covered regional cultures in each part of Thailand.

The deconstruction of both explicit and implicit meanings of sexual terms in
this book reveals the power language has to construct beliefs about gender and
sexuality. This shows that the origins of these terms lie in everyday activities that
are not intrinsically negatively loaded. It is not these activities themselves that
assign unequal value to different genders and sexual behaviors, but various societal
institutions that attempt to control sexualities, especially those of women and
people of diverse genders and sexualities. The research also demonstrates how
people attempt to create and use language in a way that assigns new meanings to
words in order to change society and to give people equal rights to express their
sexualities, while also respecting each other's rights.

INTRODUCTION TO THE ENGLISH EDITION

Peter A. Jackson

Paradoxes of Thai Sexual Culture

From a Western perspective, Thai sexual culture seems to be characterized by a number of paradoxes. On the one hand, as Niwat Kongphian observes in his preface and as all the authors of the following chapters emphasize, Thai discourses of sex and sexuality are restricted by a system of intense taboos that determine what can and cannot be said. Yet, on the other hand, as this book attests, Thai nonetheless has extraordinarily rich, varied, and multi-leveled vocabularies for the human sexual anatomy, sexual behaviors, sexual identities, and attitudes to sexuality. Indeed, in some situations, it is possible for Thai speakers to use "cute" terms for the male and female sex organs—*ju* "willy" and *jim* "fanny"—without embarrassment in contexts that would be taboo in polite circles among English speakers (N.B.: The term "fanny" is a British slang word that refers to women's genitals, unlike the American and Canadian usage of "fanny," which refers only to the buttocks).

Many foreign visitors, as well as more than a few long-term residents of Thailand, also remark on the apparent contradiction of highly visible, multi-storey "massage parlors" for well-off Thai men lining Bangkok's major thoroughfares, and the prominence of commercial sex for tourists in the city's Patpong and Soi Cowboy areas, alongside regular anti-sex tirades in the press and media orchestrated by state instrumentalities such as the Cultural Surveillance Unit within the Ministry of Culture. While some public spaces are policed to keep them sex-free ("No sex here please, we're Thai"), other nearby zones in the city are openly devoted to commodified sex for the pleasure of both heterosexual and homosexual men.

What these apparent paradoxes reflect is the high degree of contextuality of Thai cultures and discourses on sex and sexuality. In Thailand it is not sex or sex talk per se that is tabooed, but rather the revelation of the wrong images or the uttering of the wrong words at the wrong time in the wrong place. "Time and place," *kala-thesa* in Thai, that is, the social and cultural context of action, images, and speech, determines what can and cannot be said.[1] Sex talk, and for that matter sexual behavior, are not policed by a universal system of cultural prohibitions. Rather, it is the inappropriate social location or placement of discursive and visual references to eroticism that is policed and sanctioned.

For example, sex work, like sex talk, is contained within highly delimited times and places. This is made visible every evening with the dramatic cultural transition that takes place on Bangkok's Silom Road around 7 8 p.m., as the area's daytime office workers return home and the people of the night working in the area's nighttime commercial sex industry begin to arrive. This is not merely a "change of shift." It is a complete transformation of the cultural norms and expectations of this iconic downtown location in the Thai capital. The *kala-thesa*, "time and place," have changed, from daytime "sex-less" high finance and international business to nighttime commercial sex. It is the multiplicity and complexity of the sociocultural contexts of human action, and with this the many registers or levels of speech in Thai (reflected in the complexities of the Thai system of personal pronouns) that produces the apparent paradoxes of Thai sexual culture.

The Language of *Phet*:
Thailand's Master Discourse of Sex, Gender, and Sexuality

This book deals with the many dimensions of *phet*—the master discourse of sex, gender, and sexuality in modern Thai. *The Language of "Phet"* (*phasa phet*) was the title of the Thai-language version of this book. The Thai term *phet* incorporates ideas of sex, gender, and sexuality and is central to all legal, academic, as well as popular discourses of gender and sexuality. In Thai, heteronomative identities (e.g., "man," *phu-chai*; "woman," *phu-ying*) and queer subjectivities (e.g., *kathoey*, *gay*, *tom*, *dee*) are all regarded as varieties of *phet*. While all identities are imagined as blending different degrees of masculinity and femininity—and as Pimpawun Boonmongkon notes in her introduction, a gender binary underpins Thai understandings of sexual identity—the discourse of *phet* is not, as such, a binary construct. Rather, Thai discourses of *phet* reflect an understanding of

6

proliferating diversity. When Thai academics, journalists, and others write of *phet*, whether in formal or popular contexts, they typically list several, not just two, identities.

This book does not shy away from dealing directly and unflinchingly with the language for sexual physiology and sexual behavior in all its raw, sometimes humorous, often derogatory, but always colorful immediacy. It includes the registers of the spoken language (*phasa phut*), the language of the marketplace (*phasa talat*) as well as official terminologies (*phasa ratchakan*), literary usages (*phasa khian*), and technical, academic vocabularies (*phasa wichakan*). The book challenges the polite norms of Thai circumlocutions about sex by taking colloquial, earthy expressions as its analytical focus.

Key Themes: Sexual Double Standards

A key point to emerge from the following studies of Thai keywords for sex and sexuality is the intensity of the sexual double standard, with radically different normative expectations for women and men. This is another source of the apparent paradoxes of Thai sexual culture. Sexual directness in speech and openness about sexual desires and preferences are overwhelmingly male prerogatives. Almost without exception, the public contexts, or *kala-thesa*, in which sex may be talked about openly in Thailand are spaces that cater to or permit the expression of male sexual desires, whether heterosexual or homosexual. As Pimpawun and Sulaiporn Chonwilai highlight in their summary of the central findings of the Thai sexuality keywords project, and as all the other authors attest in their respective chapters, the sanctions against Thai women who are as forthright about their sexuality as Thai men regarding their desires and preferences are intense. Talking about and expressing sexual desire is seen as "natural" for heterosexual men, gays, and male-to-female transgenders and transsexuals (*kathoeys*) (and in some settings for masculine women or *toms*). However, "good" heterosexual women (*kunlasatri*) and feminine homosexual women (*dees*) are expected to remain silent about their sexuality and impassive in the face of masculine desire. Women who break these norms are denigrated and labeled as prostitutes (*sopheni*) or sluts (*dork-thorng*). An intense Madonna-whore binary structures cultural attitudes towards female sexuality.[2]

The Internet: Transgressing Thailand's Restrictive Sexual Culture

The almost exponential proliferation of Thai-language websites, chat rooms, web-boards, and e-mail lists dealing with issues of sex and sexuality, together with the use of SMS texting and mobile phones, are major phenomena of the past decade whose scope has only been outlined in the most cursory of terms by research carried out to date. In recent years, the Internet has increasingly superseded print media as the preferred medium of communication amongst younger Thai men and women. Discussions that take place on Thai-language websites are often able to evade the cultural constraints that restrict opportunities to talk openly about sex and sexuality in face-to-face contexts in everyday life. A significant part of the research for this book is based on the analysis of Thai websites, and provides fascinating insights into the new spaces for open discussion that the virtual worlds of the Thai Internet are providing in the twenty-first century. Indeed, this book reflects the ways the Internet is expanding opportunities for sexual expression among Thai people of all genders and sexualities.

Thai lesbian (*tom-dee*) culture reflects the impact of the Internet in stimulating a new wave of linguistic dynamism in the country's sexual communities in the early twenty-first century. Until recently, the single term *tom* (from "*tom*boy") has encompassed all variations of female masculinity in Thailand. However, the translator of this book, Timo Ojanen, has noted elsewhere that the binary gendering of female homosexual couples between a masculine *tom* and feminine *dee* (from "la*dy*") is being challenged, with the term *les* (abbreviated from "lesbian") now being used by women who seek to break out of gendered role play in their romantic and sexual relationships with other women.[3] The Internet is also providing a medium for younger *ying rak ying*, "women who love women," to coin a range of new labels that more appropriately reflect the gendered diversity of their lives. Young women who love women are now creating hybridized categories such as *les king* and *les queen* that draw on established notions of *gay king* (sexually active partner) and *gay queen* (sexually receptive partner) in Thai *gay* cultures to create more nuanced ways to refer to female same-sex experience and sexual preference. The ready accessibility of the Internet to younger Thais from all socioeconomic backgrounds has provided a medium to renegotiate older identity categories.

8

Critical "Queer" Perspectives on *Phet*

The authors of the following chapters analyze the language of *phet* from critical feminist and queer studies perspectives. They take the positions of women, men who love men, women who love women, and transgenders as standpoints from which to understand and critique the dominant male-centered and heteronormative structures of Thai sexual culture. The term "queer" denotes sexual and gender practices, identities, cultures, and communities that challenge normative masculine and feminine gender roles and/or transgress the borders of heterosexuality. "Queer" also labels a critical theoretical stance that analyzes all genderings and sexualities as emerging from contingent historical conditions. Queer studies views both hegemonically normative and minority genders and sexualities as interrelated components of an overarching gender/sex system in which notions of heterosexuality are constructed in relation to ideas of homosexuality, and in which understandings of transgenderism/transsexuality emerge in opposition to notions of normatively gendered and sexed behavior. This book reveals the hidden gender and sexual ideologies of mainstream ideas by reflecting on such ideas from the position of marginalized and minoritized groups. This not only reveals the diversity of these groups, it also "queers" dominant ideas. That is, it deconstructs the implicit and often hidden ideologies of mainstream discourses to reveal the sources of the cultural power of dominant ideas and concepts.

The analyses in this book are united by a shared commitment to expose, resist, and challenge the heteronormative and masculinist assumptions that marked much earlier research on Thai sexualities, and which continue to restrict the lives and opportunities of Thailand's women, *gays*, *toms*, *dees*, and *kathoeys*. The studies in the following chapters reveal how critical feminist and queer methodologies have been adopted and adapted in the twenty-first-century Thai academy to produce a powerful discourse of local critique. Indeed, this book reveals gender and sexuality in twenty-first-century Thailand to be highly contested fields.

This book also reflects the rapid expansion in Thai-language academic research on sexuality in recent years. The first Thai-language sexuality studies (*phet-withi seuksa*) conference was held in Bangkok in January 2008, with a second conference held in 2009. The chapters here showcase the path-breaking research that Thai scholars are conducting on the country's sexual cultures. Research by a new generation of Thai scholars has increasingly challenged the pathologizing, biomedical focus of much twentieth-century research on sexuality in the country.[4]

9

As Timo Ojanen has observed with respect to recent Thai research on lesbian, gay, bisexual, and transgender (LGBT) communities:

> The recent literature [on Thai LGBTs] . . . seems almost universally accepting of the sexual/gender identities of study participants; unlike earlier research, current studies no longer call for curing or preventing such identities. Today's researchers, both Thai and foreign, seem to hold that society should adapt to the needs of these minorities, rather than vice versa.[5]

While the studies here draw on an implicit queer studies methodology, the English term "queer" as such is not used in Thailand. Indeed, attempts to translate Western understandings of "queer" into Thai have had an unusual outcome and reflect the high degree of autonomy of Thai discourses of gender and sexuality with respect to international (Western) discourses. In the context of helping organize the First International Conference of Asian Queer Studies in Bangkok in July 2005, transgender-identified researcher and activist Prempreeda Pramoj Na Ayutthaya coined the compound expression *kham-phet* in an attempt to render notions of gender/sex fluidity into Thai. *Kham* means "to cross over," and Prempreeda's aim was to convey a sense of the blurring of identities within understandings of *phet*. Informed by her readings of Western queer theory, Prempreeda's neologism of *kham-phet* was an attempt to disrupt the apparent stability of the many heterosexual, same-sex, and transgender identities that are now labeled within Thai discourses of *phet*. However, *kham* is also used to translate the English prefix "trans-," as in *kham-prathet*, "transnational." Most Thai readers interpreted Prempreeda's neologism as an attempt to render the English terms "transgender" and "transsexual" into Thai, and since 2005 *kham-phet* has quickly become a generally recognized translation of these two terms, which nonetheless are not always clearly differentiated in Thai.

Prempreeda's attempt to translate "queer" into Thai quickly slipped beyond her control and became appropriated to local notions of transgenderism/transsexuality. Thai still lacks an agreed academic rendering of "queer," and authors who wish to refer to Western ideas of "queer" may write the word in roman script within their Thai texts—a common practice adopted by Thai authors when no local equivalent term is available. Hence, "queer theory" may be rendered as *tharitsadi queer*. In crossing the linguistic/discursive/cultural divide from the Anglophone West to Thailand, "queer" itself has been subjected to localized processes of queering, reflecting both the significant autonomy of

Thai discourses in representing sex/gender/sexuality, even at the height of early twenty-first-century globalization, as well as demonstrating the centrality of notions of transgenderism/transsexuality in contemporary Thai understandings of gender and sexual difference.

While Thai lacks a precise local rendering of "queer," terms for "gender" and "sexuality" have been coined. Since the 1990s, the English term "gender" has been variously rendered as *sathanaphap thang-phet*, *phet-sathan*, *phet-phawa*, *phet-saphap*, and *phet-saphawa* (all denoting "*phet* condition" or "*phet* status"), with *phet-phawa* emerging as a commonly accepted translation among Thai feminist academics. Over the past decade, the term "sexuality" has been translated as *phet-withi* ("*phet* orientation"). The authors of this book all use *phet-phawa* for "gender" and *phet-withi* for "sexuality."

Given the diversity and dynamism of Thai *gay*, lesbian, and transgender terminologies, Thai academics and LGBT activists have struggled to find an agreed overarching term for all the country's genders and sexualities. The need for such a common term emerged in 2007 with the formation of a united front of lesbians, *gays*, and *kathoeys* to lobby the Thai government on a range of human rights issues. These efforts focused on attempts to enshrine an anti-discrimination clause in the Thai constitution, to permit male-to-female transgenders and transsexuals to have their feminine status recognized on identity cards and passports, and to overturn the Thai army's definition of *kathoey* conscripts as mentally ill. Since 2007, the expression *khwam-lak-lai thang-phet*, which in different contexts can be rendered variously as "gender/sexual diversity" or "diverse genders/sexualities," has emerged as the banner under which Thailand's diverse queer communities have come together in common political cause and remains the closest Thai equivalent to Western understandings of "queer." The language of "queer rights" has been translated formally into Thai as *sitthi khorng khon thi mi khwam-lak-lai thang-phet*, literally "the rights of people who possess *phet*-diversity." In this book the phraseology "people of diverse sexualities and genders" has been used to translate *khon thi mi khwam-lak-lai thang-phet*, an expression that this book's authors use frequently.

Successful Discursive Activism
by Thai Feminist and Queer NGOs and Academics

The range of feminist- and queer-inspired neologisms for sex, gender, and sexuality detailed above reflects a little-recognized success story of civil society activism in Thailand over the past two decades. Thai feminist and LGBT activists and academics have put considerable energy into lobbying the bureaucracy and counteracting negative media stereotyping, and have been remarkably successful in challenging discriminatory and pathologizing mainstream terminologies and discourses. Thai LGBT activists have identified pathologizing stereotyping in both visual media and public discourses as key sources of the ongoing discrimination suffered by queer people in the country. In response, Thai people of diverse genders and sexualities have pursued strategies of cultural activism to resist and supplant the pathologizing stereotypes that pervade the domains of visual and discursive representation.

The lesbian NGO Anjaree and feminist academic supporters in several Thai universities initiated this discursive activism in the 1990s, and together they have been singularly influential in changing the languaging of *gay*, lesbian, and transgender issues in the bureaucracy, electronic media, broadsheet newspapers, and weekly news review magazines. There has been less success in changing the often lurid, discriminatory language used in mass-circulation popular daily newspapers such as *Thai Rath* and *Daily News*, which continue to use derogatory terms such as *tut* (effeminate faggot) on front-page news banner headlines.

The discursive shifts achieved by this activism are reflected in the table on the next page and represent the dramatic qualitative change in the languaging of sexuality issues in the Thai academy and in mainstream press and media reporting that has taken place as a direct result of concerted feminist and queer activism. Pimpawun Boonmongkon has been a key player in this discursive activism, with the Center for Health Policy Studies that she heads at Mahidol University being a key institutional base for critical feminist and queer studies research in Thailand. In his own research, Timo Ojanen has found that Thai sexual/gender categories, labels, and analytic terms "are being consciously developed [both within the communities and amongst academics] and adapted to improve the status of each minority group."[6] All the authors here conduct their analyses within the critical frame of the new non-discriminatory and inclusive terminologies that Thailand's discursive activists have struggled to develop in recent years.

Changing Thai Discourses of Gender/Sex Diversity

Before 2000: Pathologizing, Discriminatory Terminologies[a]	
rak-ruam-phet	homosexuality (biomedical)
wiparit thang-phet	sexually perverted (psychiatric, moralistic)
biang-ben thang-phet	sex/gender deviant (biomedical)
After 2000: New Non-Discriminatory, Inclusive Terminologies[b]	
phet-phawa	gender (lit. "*phet* status/condition")
phet-withi	sexuality (lit. "the path/direction of *phet*," i.e., sexual orientation)
kham-phet	transgender (lit. "crossing over *phet*")
rak phet-diao-kan	same-sex love (lit. "love of the same *phet*;" used in place of *rak-ruam-phet*)
khwam-lak-lai thang-phet	gender/sex diversity (lit. "*phet* diversity")
ying rak ying	women who love women (used in place of "lesbian")
chai rak chai	men who love men (used in place of *chai rak-ruam-phet*)
sao praphet sorng	transgender (lit. "second type of woman;" used in place of *tut*, etc.)

[a] These terms have been critiqued and rejected by this volume's authors.
[b] This volume's authors use these terms instead.

Globalization and Thailand's Twenty-First-Century Sexual Cultures

Despite the presence of large numbers of Western tourists, the circulation of dubbed and subtitled Western movies, and the reproduction (often via unlicensed pirating) of Western pornography and images from Western magazines, the relationship between Thailand's sexual cultures and the West cannot be categorized in simplistic terms as either "neocolonial" cultural imperialism or "postcolonial resistance." As Rachel Harrison and I have noted elsewhere, the fact that Thailand was never colonized by a Western power places this society in an ambiguous relationship to accounts of Euro-American imperialism.[7] Internationally circulating Western discourses of sexuality, homosexuality, gayness, queer, and so on have not led to unmediated "cultural borrowing" of

Western sexualities in Thailand so much as a new repertoire of ways to retell local stories, and alternative ways to remember local histories.

As Fran Martin et al. point out in a comparative study of queer cultural developments across East and Southeast Asia, notions of cultural hybridity that foreground the power of local agency and the resilience of local discourses provide a more fruitful lens for conceptualizing what has been happening in Asian sexual cultures, including Thailand, over recent decades.[8] The fascinating detailed studies here of twenty-one keywords of modern Thai understandings of *phet* reflect the fact that while Thailand continues to become more intimately integrated into global economic and cultural networks, the country's sexual cultures nonetheless exhibit a remarkable distinctiveness. Accurately understanding the specificity of Thai discourses and cultures of *phet* can only take place once we possess a non-discriminatory vocabulary that represents all the country's diverse genders and sexualities as equal. This book provides a vital foundation for the further development of Thai sexuality studies in the years ahead.

KEY FINDINGS

Sulaiporn Chonwilai
Pimpawun Boonmongkon

Here, we provide a general overview of our research findings, analyzing the power of language to create discourses, or so-called social "truths," about sexual matters and the involvement of various societal institutions in reproducing and legitimizing such discourses as mainstream truths or knowledge. Neutral sexual terminology that reflects spoken language dealing with sexual matters as a part of everyday life is also presented. Finally, the creation and use of language in the context of appropriate social space and power is also dealt with following Norman Fairclough, who asserts that whether the value of certain expressions increases or decreases depends on the power the language user has.[1]

Language-Directed Sexual Matters

Language used to discuss sexual topics not only describes its object, but also reflects the background of the language user in terms of gender, age, social class, wealth, education, and locale, as well as the norms, values, and belief systems of the society and culture within which the language is used. Sexual terminology has various registers, such as the everyday spoken language of ordinary people (whose usage might at times appear coarse and impolite), language favored by the media, youth, and other types of slang, formal language, and medical jargon.

Thai sexual vocabularies include older terms that are still in use, as well as more recent ones that communicate new perspectives about sexual matters and constitute a contestation of the meanings of old, prejudiced terms that reflect sexual inequalities. Contemporary Thai sexual language also contains borrowed English terms, which suggests that the sexual behaviors such terms describe may have not previously been in the open in Thai society or are based on Western values, and thus have not previously had descriptive labels in Thai.

In this study, the meanings of words are analyzed from a deconstructionist viewpoint, which holds that words do not have fixed, inherent meanings. Rather, they form a part of a web of meanings within the structure of language. Besides having a direct meaning (denotation), every term also has implied meanings (connotations) that differ from the direct meaning. The meanings of words are thus fluid and change from one context to another. For example, the word *kathoey* can refer to a seedless fruit as well an intersex or transsexual person. In the past, it referred to both transgendered males and females, but is now only used for those who are born with male anatomy but who express femininity via their external appearance and behavior.

Language is a crucial medium in the reproduction of meanings and the associated transmission of sexual values from one generation of language users to the next. Sexual terminology is thus very influential in shaping perspectives, beliefs, understandings, and so-called knowledge on sexual matters.

The analysis of the twenty-one keywords in this book indicates that Thai beliefs on sexual matters can be summarized as follows.

A Dominant System of Two Sexes:
Two Genders and One Normative Sexuality

Like most other societies, Thai society believes that there are only two "natural" human sexes: male (*phet-chai*) and female (*phet-ying*), and that these are determined by the person's sex organs, known by various names (e.g., *hee*, *jim*, *hoi*, etc., for the female sex organs; *khuay*, *jiao*, *ham*, etc., for the male sex organs). Persons with other types of sex organs (e.g., those with both female and male, or indeterminate sex organs) are seen as abnormal and no terms exist for the specific character of their sex organs. The same holds true for the sex organs of persons who have had sex reassignment surgery.

Just as in the case of physiological sexes, Thai society also divides genders into two types, man (*phu-chai*) and woman (*phu-ying*), generally regarded as being linked to the person's sex organs. That is, a person born with female sex organs is expected to have a feminine gender identity and feminine characteristics, e.g., dress in a feminine way, have feminine manners, have a "natural" maternal instinct, be soft and weak, have a lower sex drive than men, and be the receptive/

passive party in sex. In contrast, a person born with male sex organs is expected to have a masculine gender identity and characteristics, e.g., dress in a masculine way, be strong and a natural leader, have a higher sex drive than women, and be the insertive/active party in sex. A person born with one set of genitalia, but who expresses a gender not usually associated with that set of genitalia, is not accepted and is stigmatized as abnormal. The same is true for those whose gender does not fall neatly into either of the two gender categories.

This dominant system accepts only one type of normative sexuality, which is comprised of *a heterosexual orientation, sexual desire toward the opposite sex, and heterosexual sex for the purpose of procreation.* Furthermore, only vaginal penetration by a penis is seen as normal, natural sex. Desiring or having sex with a person of one's own sex, anal sex, oral sex (homosexual or heterosexual), and masturbation are all seen as sexual practices outside society's framework and/or as abnormal.

Valuing Masculinity More Than Femininity

In this dominant ideological system of two normative sexes, two genders, and one sexuality, societal expectations and socialization processes are different for men and women. Men are expected to be leaders and women the followers in every issue, including but not limited to sexual matters.

Men are believed to have a higher sex drive and a higher need for sexual outlets than women. This belief system gives men the freedom to learn about and have access to sexual matters and also to have various types of sex with various types of people, without being condemned as harshly as is the case for women. Women, on the other hand, still have to be chaste (*rak nuan sa-nguan tua*) and abide by what society defines as the characteristics of a "good woman." For example, a woman should not dress in a revealing, sexually provocative way (*po*) in public, because this is seen as inviting men to sexually harass or to commit sexual violence against her. In addition to this, a woman must not have sex before marriage, show interest in sex, or behave in the way referred to as being *Khun Phaen*, that is, a womanizer, in the case of men. Women who do so are considered "bad women" and are variously branded as *raet, ran, Kaki, Wanthorng*, or with some other stigmatizing term.

Women are also expected to get married and have children to be considered complete women. Those who have not married by the age Thai women usually do are subjected to malicious gossip that insinuates something must be wrong with them. It is assumed that no man wants to marry them, and so they are said to have become spinsters (*kheun khan*).

Male supremacy over women in sexual matters is particularly visible within heterosexual sexualities, in which men are expected to be sexual experts, sexually experienced, the active/insertive party in sex, and the leader in sexual matters. In these contexts, the main objective of sex is the man's achievement of orgasm (*set*) or ejaculation. Some men think that the woman's achievement of *set* also depends on the man's experience and expertise in sex, rather than any role the woman may play in sex. The supposedly male-only emotion of sex obsession (*heun*), the production and consumption of pornographic materials (*seu po*) to stimulate male sex drives, and buying services from prostitutes (*sopheni*) are all aspects of a male-centered sexual culture.

Patriarchal values also influence homosexual sexualities, which are similar to heterosexual ones in that the party adopting a masculine role (whether a *tom* in the case of women who love women or a *gay king* in the case of men who love men) communicates it by clothing, gender expressions, and being the active/insertive party in sex. Some women who love women and who assume gendered roles (i.e., a masculine *tom* and a feminine *dee*) view womanizing *toms* like they would view a womanizing man or *Khun Phaen*.

Values of Monogamy and Sex Based on Love

Thai society believes that a good sexuality is one that operates within a lasting monogamous relationship, is based on love (not on sexual pleasure alone), and involves no *swinging* (partner swapping). Society authorizes such relationships through traditions and the marriage institution. Other types of sex (e.g., sex for money, *swinging*, etc.) or having a casual partner (*kik*) are seen as "bad."

Sex Is (Supposed to Be) Only for Procreation

The Thai ideals regarding sexual life involve valuing sex for procreation more than for pleasure. Any sexuality that does not involve this perpetuation of the family and the creation of new citizens for the country, such as sex between persons who love the same sex, commercial sex, *swinging*, anal or oral sex, and masturbation, is seen as having lower value, deviating from society's standards, being abnormal, and requiring treatment or eradication from society.

These mainstream Thai ideals are supported by religious teachings, culture, traditions, societal practices, medicine, and psychology. Hence, those who think differently or have a gender identity or sexuality that differs from such ideals are judged as being outside of society's framework, are not accepted, and are possibly stigmatized as sexually deviant or as a social problem that has to be corrected or punished for setting a bad example for society's youth.

Neutrality and Ordinariness in Sexual Language

Many sexual terms are neutral, considered neither dirty nor vulgar, nor as an instrument of sexual oppression. For example, *ao kan*, *eup kan*, and *pi kan* are used informally between friends, and all connote consensuality of having sex, as does *mi sek*, which is similar, if somewhat more formal and broader in meaning. In contrast to these, *dai sia* and *sia tua* connote sexual inequality, implying that the woman "loses" and the man "gains"—or at least does not lose his reputation—from the sexual act.

Neutral terms exist also for female sexual physiology, for example *jim*, *khoey*, or *pet* (the last two are Southern Thai terms). Even *hee* (cunt) is quite neutral, not obscene, when used by rural people or by transsexual *kathoey*. For example, a *kathoey* may say, "Let me have a look at your *hee*," when asking another *kathoey* friend to show the results of her sex reassignment surgery. The widespread use of the word *kik* (casual partner) by people of almost all genders and ages also suggests that temporary or polyamorous relations are increasingly seen as normal.

The Power of Language in Changing Sexual Culture

However intensely the state attempts to force its subjects' sexualities into a mainstream framework, those who do not share a belief in the mainstream gender/sexuality ideology and those with non-mainstream gender identities and sexualities, nevertheless, attempt to create spaces for expressing their sexual desires and identities. They negotiate and challenge state power, either within their own small groups or by uniting in activism to make the violations of their sexual rights known to the state, to present new perspectives on gender and sexuality, to increase acceptance of their group, and to reduce sexual prejudice against themselves. The creation of terms like *ying rak ying* (women who love women), *chai rak chai* (men who love men) and *phanak-ngan borikan* ("service worker" as a euphemism for a sex worker) shows how language can be used to deconstruct the meanings of old, prejudiced terms like *lesbian* (which has negative connotations in Thai), *chai rak-ruam-phet* (a male homosexual) and *sopheni* (a prostitute), respectively. Another example is analysis of the word *hee* (cunt), which uncovers the exercise of power and sexual oppression concealed within both the meaning and usage of words for women's sexual organs. The use of alternative terms like *trong nan*, *khorng sa-nguan*, or *thi lap* for the female sex organs reflects resistance to the sort of oppression of women that debases them by linking them with the negative connotations of terms used for the sex organs.

A System of Two Genders and One Normative Sexuality: Power and Implications for Sexual Rights and Sexual Health

The more society tries to make sexual matters taboo by restricting them to the private sphere, the more they are talked about, consumed, or dealt with by means of gossip. In addition to attempting to uncover the origins of the mainstream Thai belief system on gender and sexuality, our research team has also tried to bring the resulting problems, namely, sexual ill-being, into the open. This includes stigmatization, rights violations, violence against those with non-mainstream genders or sexualities (e.g., people who love the same sex, sex workers, etc.), or the higher value given to men than women in sexual matters. Our team has also highlighted where Thailand's reproductive health or sexual health services fail to meet the needs of service users due to the providers' lack of understanding and awareness of sexual and gender diversity.

All of these problems result from assumptions, attitudes, values, and knowledge on sexual matters that are locked into the ideological system of two normative genders and one normative sexuality, and which reject other gender and sexuality systems. Such perspectives are similar to the belief that any given word has a single, inherent meaning (while other, similar meanings are excluded). These perspectives retain their currency despite the diversity of gender and sexual identities found in contemporary Thai society, which is demonstrated by the increasing public presence of other gender and sexual identity groups such as *sao praphet sorng* (transgender individuals) and people who love the same sex.

Furthermore, gender and sexual identity are not fixed characteristics. They are fluid and ever changing, which shows that they are socially constructed and not determined from birth. For example, terms related to the word *kathoey*, like *sao praphet sorng* (lit. "second type of woman") or *sao siap* (lit. "penetrating girl"), reflect attempts to deconstruct the societal perception of all *kathoeys* as being a homogeneous group. Researchers have pointed to the diversity found in the sexual practices and external characteristics of *kathoeys*. Likewise, the expression *chai rak chai* is related to a group of other terms—including *gay queen*, *gay king*, and *gay both*—which show that sexual practices among men who love men are dependent on the context of the relationship rather than being fixed.

The hegemony of the mainstream sexuality discourse in controlling people's sexuality-related beliefs and sexual practices is due to the state's attempts to control and shape people's sexual lives through various societal mechanisms. These include the creation of "truths" on sexual matters (validated with medical or psychological explanations), the creation of sexual values (legitimized by reference to morals or religious commandments), perspectives on birth control, and various legal principles. In other words, the mainstream sexuality discourse does not operate on its own. Rather, it is a part of a socially constructed web of truths and knowledge on sexual matters, which are produced, shaped, and disseminated through societal mechanisms. For example, consider medicine's past view of loving the same sex (homosexuality) as supposedly being a sexual abnormality. When it was finally revealed there was no clear empirical evidence to support this theory, medical and psychological circles, in the end, announced the removal of homosexuality from the mental disorder classification scheme and treatment manuals. However, while academic understandings of homosexuality have already changed, most people still view homosexuality as an abnormality (because it transgresses societal values on sexual matters) or as a sin (because it violates religious injunctions).

Similarly, anal and oral sex are nowadays viewed in a more positive light as matters of personal taste and/or a person's right to his or her own body. Yet many people still consider these practices as abnormal activities, with the argument that the anus and the mouth are not naturally designed for sex and that only two men having sex together have to resort to them, being unable to have so-called normal, penetrative sex.

Masturbation, which is considered as having less value than penetrative sex, is given different explanations for men and women. For men, it is seen as a natural venting of sexual pressure, although penetrative sex would still be preferable. In contrast, society assumes that women should be able to control themselves and not express their sexual feelings, unless a man invites them to do so first. Failing this, they may be seen as not being "good women" (*kunlasatri*).

While society tells its members that sexual matters are private, certain kinds of sexual relations that would seem to be especially private, such as swapping partners (*swinging*), sex in exchange for money (i.e., with *sopheni*), casual sex with several people (*kik* relations), or the consumption of porn (*seu po*), are seen as behaviors dangerous to society, which justifies the state's attempt to eradicate them in order to maintain the existing moral order.

Not only those with non-mainstream gender or sexual identities face pressure in sexual matters. People with mainstream identities, that is, gender-normative heterosexual men and women are also governed by the mainstream sexuality discourse, which influences their practices and ways of thinking in subtle ways. This is particularly true for the gender most deprived of selfhood and sexual rights, i.e., women.

Thai society has high expectations for women, namely, that they will be chaste loyal wives, good mothers, and homemakers who pursue housekeeping to perfection. They are expected to maintain their virginity/hymen (the same word, *phrommajan*, is used for both in Thai) until they give it to a man they love and marry; be chaste (*rak nuan sa-nguan tua*) before marriage; neither talk about nor show any interest in sexual matters; not reveal their sexual desires or take initiative in sexual matters; not dress in a sexually provocative (*po*) way; not love or have sex with other women; and not remain single, because that would constitute *kheun khan*—becoming a spinster—and signal their lack of ideal feminine characteristics, which would, in turn, mean no man would want to look at them. Finally, their value is measurable in money, through the bride price (*sin sort*) payable to their parents by the bridegroom prior to marriage. This means women are still expected to abide by traditional values of respect, obedience, and gratitude toward their parents. In other words, they still lack true freedom to make their own choices in life.

But men also face expectations from society. They are supposed to have strong sex drives and to act as leaders in every matter (e.g., family, sex). While, on the one hand, their consumption of pornographic materials and the *kheun khru* ceremony of sexual initiation (see chapter 14) reflect their sexual freedom, on the other hand, these constitute propping up masculinity in order to build credibility and acceptance within male peer groups. Men who do not meet societal expectations for their masculinity, such as those who wear women's clothes, have sex change operations, love other men, engage in non-mainstream sexual behaviors (e.g., anal sex, *swinging*), or are sexually impotent are castigated and stigmatized just like those who have non-mainstream genders or sexualities. Nevertheless, both heterosexual and homosexual men have more freedom to express their sexual desires than women do.

The main objective of this study is not to create new definitions for sexual terms, but rather to analyze such terms from the perspectives of gender and sexuality, in order to examine the mainstream sexuality discourse that underpins them (and their usage) as well as to demonstrate the power language has to shape people's sexual practices and ways of thinking about sexual matters. Both language and sexual matters are constructed through complex and subtle societal mechanisms. Meanings conveyed by language can shift or be interpreted in various ways, depending on the sociocultural context and who exactly is using what language to communicate with whom. The power of language in directing beliefs in sexual matters is based on its role in transmitting the mainstream sexuality discourse from one generation to the next. This discourse is linked to many societal problems and the ways in which people try to solve them, such as inequality between men and women, oppression and discrimination against people who have non-mainstream genders and sexualities, and sexual violence.

One of the main messages of this study is that the mainstream belief system of sexual matters in Thailand affects sexual health, as people do not always fall into the expectations and roles laid out by this belief system. In fact, people manifest genders and engage in sexual practices that resist and challenge the power of this dominant discourse. When such people face sexual health problems and need to address them through services provided by the state, and if the perspectives and normative expectations of the staff of such services do not match the sexuality and gender identity of the service users, their needs will not be effectively met. This is because the service users may not dare to tell the staff openly about the origins of their problems, or may face discrimination from staff that are prejudiced against such client groups.

In our era, women and men are more equal than before. Many more women have educational opportunities, economic independence, and more freedom to express themselves sexually than in the past. Groups of homosexual people are able to be more public than before. Sex change technologies are available for those with the financial means to afford them. With advancements in information technology, pornographic materials are now available in every format, covering sexual activities satisfying every taste and relationship type. Yet our apparently sexually tolerant society still encounters numerous sex-related problems, such as virulent STDs, various reproductive health issues, sexual violence, and hatred and oppression of those with non-mainstream sexualities and genders.

This analysis of sex-related terminology is an attempt to review, examine, and pose questions regarding the Thai belief system on sexual matters, such as: "How does Thai society really view sexual matters?" and "Do we really have freedom in sexual matters?" This was done by choosing language as the object of analysis and by trying to deconstruct the dominant mainstream belief system in sexual matters to reveal the sexual prejudices that we all harbor. The ultimate object of this research is to build a society characterized by sexual health, in which people of all gender identities and sexualities can happily coexist and be equal with one another, and in which friendly and supportive sexual health services that meet the needs of people of all gender identities and sexualities are provided.

PART 1

DOMINANT CULTURAL ATTITUDES TO SEXUALITY

1 *REUANG PHET* (เรื่องเพศ): SEXUAL MATTERS

Monruedee Laphimon

About *Phet*: Language and the Shaping of Power

Phet (เพศ) is one of the most difficult Thai words to define because this term, derived from Sanskrit (*vesha* เวษ) and Pali (*vesa* เวส), has a very broad meaning, ranging from the anatomical differences between males and females through to the emotions, feelings, and desires that define masculinity and femininity, including sexual activities and behaviors. In 1984, several debates arose among the members of the committee charged with preparing the new, revised version of the *Royal Institute Dictionary* when they attempted to define the word *phet*. In the 1982 edition, the word had been defined tersely: "*phet* n., the distinguishing form (*rup* รูป) of femaleness or maleness; (grammar) a word category in Pali, Sanskrit, etc., equivalent to *ling* (ลิงถ์) or *leung* (ลึงค์) [i.e., grammatical gender]."[1] In 1984, the meaning of "the distinguishing form of femaleness or maleness" in the first part of the definition was contested. Finally, the committee agreed on a new definition for the word *phet*, as follows:

> ***phet***: n., [in humans] the characteristics (*rupalaksana* รูปลักษณะ) that distinguish women (*ying*) from men (*chai*), as in the words *satri-phet* (สตรีเพศ), "female sex," *burut-phet* (บุรุษเพศ), "male sex;" in animals, the characteristics that distinguish the male (*tua-phu*) from the female (*tua-mia*), as in the words *phet-phu* (เพศผู้), the "male sex," *phet-mia* (เพศเมีย), the "female sex;" the characteristics or common practices that distinguish a group, e.g., *samana-phet* (สมณเพศ), the "status of an ordained Buddhist monk," *khihi-phet* (คิหิเพศ), the "lay status of a householder," *phet-khareuhat* (เพศคฤหัสถ์), the "status of a lay person," *phet-banphachit* (เพศบรรพชิต), the "status of an ordained priest or monk;" (grammar) a word category in Pali, Sanskrit, etc., equivalent to *ling* (ลิงค์) or *leung* (ลึงค์) [i.e., grammatical gender].[2]

27

Although the revised definition was broader than the former one, it still lacked clarity because the meanings of some related terms were not clearly specified, such as *kitjakam thang-phet* (กิจกรรมทางเพศ), "sexual activity," *khwam-samphan thang-phet* (ความสัมพันธ์ทางเพศ), "sexual relationships" or "sexual relations," *kan-ruam-phet* (การร่วมเพศ), "to engage in sexual intercourse," *khwam-ruseuk thang-phet* (ความรู้สึกทางเพศ), "sexual feelings," or *phetsarot* (เพศรส), "sexual tastes." It was thus agreed that another word that would cover such meanings be added; namely, *kam* (กาม), "eroticism/sex" or *kamarom* (กามารมณ์), "sexual feelings," thus replacing *phet* with *kam*. However, the committee did not provide definitions for *phet-sat* (เพศศาสตร์), "sexology," or *phet-seuksa* (เพศศึกษา), "sex education" or "studies in sex."[3]

This reflects the roots of how the current way of thinking about sexual matters and the meanings given words associated with sexual matters in Thai society are shaped through the use of language and choices of wording. The shaping of the definition of the word *phet* by the Royal Institute began with a very narrowly defined term that came directly from Pali and Sanskrit words that dealt with sexual organs, such as *awaiyawa phet* (อวัยวะเพศ) and *khreuang phet* (เครื่องเพศ), or reproductive organs, such as *awaiyawa seup-phan* (อวัยวะสืบพันธุ์). The word *phet* was seen in terms of binary opposites—male vs. female—that constitute the main indicators of anatomical sex and a set of conditions for the expression of masculine and feminine gender roles. More recently, further development has led to the following four-pronged official definition:

- an individual's way of leading his/her everyday life linked to his/her involvement with or rejection of sexual matters;
- the dimension of sexual feelings and emotions;
- sexual relations; and
- sexual practices/behaviors.

Matters Below the Belly Button: Sexual Matters and Their Contested Meanings

Words and phrases related to *phet* can be divided into two main groups: those that reflect a conservative, negative perception of sexual matters as lowly and base, such as *reuang tai sadeu* (เรื่องใต้สะดือ), "matters below the belly button," *reuang yang wa* (เรื่องอย่างว่า), "that kind of thing/those kinds of things," *reuang nai mung* (เรื่องในมุ้ง), "matters within the mosquito net," and *reuang bon tieng* (เรื่องบนเตียง),

28

"matters in the bed;" and those that reflect neutral or positive perceptions of sexual activity as a matter of rights or the subject of education, such as *reuang sek* (เรื่องเซ็กส์), *reuang phet* (เรื่องเพศ), and *reuang thang-phet* (เรื่องทางเพศ), all three of which literally denote "sexual matters."

Words in the first group reflect sexual matters as shameful, harmful, scandalous, or evil, linking them to depravity and sexual violence. This is represented in the use of the idiom *reuang tai sadeu*, "matters below the belly button," as in the following headings and postings on various Internet news sites:

- Weird statue in a Korean park smacks a bit of *reuang tai sadeu*.[4]
- Another scandal in MoSDHS [Ministry of Social Development and Human Security]! *Reuang tai sadeu* revealed as provincial chief sexually violates, gropes his female subordinate's bum for years.[5]
- While other political parties are brainstorming about ways to solve the country's problems, politicians in some parties only think about *reuang tai sadeu* or tricks by which to destroy the constitution that most people in the country accept.[6]

Reuang tai sadeu describes sexual activities or behavior, and reflects sexual matters as private. Related terms may also convey the place and time in which sexual activities take place among different social groups. The idioms *reuang yang wa*, "that kind of thing," *reuang nai mung*, "matters inside the mosquito net," and *reuang bon tiang*, "matters in bed," reflect the different ways of life in urban and rural settings, whether communicating about the modern practice of sleeping in a bed or the traditional ways of sleeping on the floor and having to use a mosquito net to cover the bed. All these idioms are common in popular media and on the Internet, as seen from the following examples from various websites:

- *Reuang yang wa* that women want to ask about.[7]
- Hello. I am also a person who likes *reuang yang wa* a lot. It makes me feel like I'm not a good elder sibling (*phi*) for my younger siblings (*norng-norng*). It will probably remain as a stigma on me for the rest of my life. But I don't think it's that wrong . . .[8]
- *Reuang bon tiang* that young women don't want.[9]
- I am a person who enjoys *reuang bon tiang* without realizing it. I married my husband when I was still young. My husband was thirty-five and I was just twenty-two. In the past, we lived in Bangkok, just the two of us . . .[10]
- Baem & Bo clarify *reuang nai mung*: tell about the "same husband" scandal.[11]

Expressions within the second group, such as *reuang phet* or *reuang sek,* reflect explanations of sexual matters from a more neutral and/or academic, medical, social, or sexual rights perspective. They also relate to sexual belief systems and sexual education.

The expression *reuang phet* is used in academic and official texts that relate to beliefs and meanings concerning sexual matters. It is also used in campaigns that aim to change the sexual values that are at the root of society's sexual standards, as in the following post to a website that discussed an officially-sponsored sex education camp for school-age teenagers:

> The previous facilitator added that activities in this camp were of the type called "activities for trendsetting," that is, besides working with people who work with young people in schools, societal understanding on *reuang phet* has to be built [so that people understand] that they are not just matters of sexual intercourse, but their context is that of life, learning from birth to death . . .[12]

Reuang phet is used in publications that involve learning, awareness, and access to information as well as in unbiased, comprehensive sexual counseling to reduce negative sexual health outcomes, as in the following section taken from a Ministry of Public Health publication:

> Awareness of *reuang phet* involves information, facts, beliefs, experiences . . . Beliefs influence our expressions. *Phet is a natural matter of life*; everyone must have correct knowledge and understanding of *reuang phet*. Don't believe anything easily, but use reason and facts, too, because if it's a correct reality, it will be explainable by scientific principles. People tend to practise according to their beliefs. Thus, if we believe in something that's not right, not good, not appropriate, it might be bad for our health or be harmful to us, make us behave in a way that is risky for our health; for example, the belief that "if a woman rushes to urinate and wash after intercourse, it will protect against pregnancy" can put women at risk of STDs and AIDS.[13]

Reuang phet is also used in discussions about sexual freedom and equality between the sexes, as in the following post by a woman to a web discussion on whether women should speak openly about their sexual experiences:

I think it depends on whether you can repress these things or not. And if yes, it'll probably be good to be open and release one's feelings verbally. But I feel that it might not be that necessary. Divulging *reuang phet* and achieving sexual equality (*khwam-thao-thiam thang-phet*) aren't the same thing. Even if tomorrow we women could be totally open about *reuang phet*, the old problem of sexual inequality would still not go away. So, what good is it?[14]

Reuang phet, or "sexual matters," includes sexual pleasure, feelings, needs, satisfaction, and ability, as seen in the following quote from a magazine's advice column:

Dear Reader, did you know that problems of *reuang phet*, such as frigidity, lack of satisfaction in sex, reduced sexual libido, premature ejaculation, inability to have an ejaculation during intercourse, not reaching a climax, impotence, the woman feeling pain during sex or muscle stiffness in the vaginal area, are all caused by mental problems? There are a few other causes . . .[15]

Sek (เซ็กส์) is borrowed from the English word "sex," but its sense in Thai differs from the English one. It was only recently added to the *Royal Institute Dictionary of New Words:*

sek: n. (1) sexual need, as in "That guy's *sek jat* (เซ็กส์จัด—sexually hyperactive). Watch out when you're near him;" (2) sexual intercourse, as in "Elders should teach kids not to have *sek* when they're still young;" (3) sexual provocation, as in "Children should not be allowed to read Japanese comic books too much. They're all full of *sek*."

sek: v. to attract the opposite sex, as in "The latest guy was so *sek* . . . [I'd] go [with him] straight away" or "This woman dresses the most *sek* in the event" (means the same as sexy).[16]

The word *sek* is yet another Thai term that has quite a broad meaning and can be used in several contexts, whether in everyday speech or in formal use, as in the following quotes from a safe sex information website and a newspaper article, respectively:

- Twenty women's *reuang sek* problems—solved (simple *reuang sek* matters that men don't know).[17]
- What makes it so visually appealing and exciting is the use of materials like condoms or contraceptive pills as instructional equipment, which are really the same as when Social Studies uses country maps and science classes have experiments. As for the criticism, let me say that you've got to see it to its end to do justice to it. If we don't teach kids to understand what *reuang phet, reuang sek* are like, then what's going to happen? If you really can't bear it, then don't send your kids to study here, teach them at home like you did in the past.[18]

The above examples show that *reuang phet* as a term is neutral and lends itself to being used with various issues, such as sexual rights and equality, sexual pleasure and satisfaction, diversity, gender and sexuality differences, and so on. All of this comes from the attempts of various groups to contribute to defining what *reuang phet* means. This can be based on anatomical differences, as in the past, or by redefining sexual matters positively, as a natural thing for people of all genders, who should have the freedom to choose how to find their own path to sexual pleasure.

The Power of Academic Knowledge and its Health Implications

Traditional perspectives that view *reuang phet* negatively prevent groups like children, youth, and women from accessing impartial information on sexual matters. Among the most closely watched groups are young men and women. This can be seen from numerous studies on *reuang phet* among youth that are produced by both public and private bodies concerned about youth sexual behavior. These studies often express fear that young people will become sex addicts. Both medical doctors and psychologists have volunteered information on how sexual addiction among youth is linked to frequent masturbation or sex, having several partners, having high sexual needs, giving importance to sex, looking at pornographic books, viewing pornographic cartoons or videos, talking about sexual needs with friends, telling sexually loaded anecdotes, and so on.[19]

Recent studies by the Institute for Population and Social Research at Mahidol University, including a 2005 survey on youth attitudes on life and love, a 2006 report on the health situation of children, youth, and families, and a 2007 report on sexual matters among youth aged eighteen to nineteen, as well as national reports on the AIDS situation perpetuate the mainstream perspective on monitoring and controlling risky sexual behavior among youth. This information is legitimized by medical knowledge but also reflects the population science perspective, which focuses on the population's so-called quality and safety, as seen in statements like "making Thailand the country with the highest rate of births among people younger than nineteen in Southeast Asia."

All of this contradicts traditional beliefs about children and youth being sexually innocent, which greatly affects the selection of content to be presented in youth sex education programs. This is often due to the fear that giving information too openly amounts to the same thing as telling youth to have sex even earlier. Society has thus campaigned and devised ways of controlling youth sexualities in every way, to protect children and youth from *reuang phet* and to attempt to decrease their interest in sex. Psychological and moralistic knowledge has been used to make children feel guilty and afraid when involved with sexual matters. There have been attempts to instill the societal ideal of chastity or *rak nuan sa-nguan tua* in youth (see chapter 2), and there has also been stigmatization of youth involved with sexual matters as evidenced in the terms *dek tit sek* (เด็กติด เซ็กส์), "sex-addicted kids" and *dek jai-taek* (เด็กใจแตก), "problem kids." This type of disparaging labeling of youth sexualities by state authorities can be considered to be a form of violence against children and youth. Furthermore, these approaches do not solve sexual problems in a youth-centered way.

However, it is not just young people who are seen as having sexual problems. The mainstream framework for sexuality limits, controls, and oppresses people's sexualities regardless of their gender or age. It also affects the provision of sexual health services, within which the diversity of genders and sexualities is insufficiently considered. All this is due to the role of "facts" produced by medical experts, linguists, lexicographers, and population scientists that often reproduce negative beliefs that bind *reuang phet* and *reuang sek* within a narrow gender/ sexuality frame (e.g., a belief that sex should take place only within a heterosexual, monogamous marriage for procreation, or the belief that only adults should learn about sexual matters). As long as this conservative framework remains unanalyzed and unquestioned, society will continue, as it has in the past, to see problems of what it considers sexual ill-being.

2 *RAK NUAN SA-NGUAN TUA* (รักนวลสงวนตัว): TO BE CHASTE

Monruedee Laphimon

A Popular Mantra for Controlling Female Sexuality

Rak nuan sa-nguan tua (รักนวลสงวนตัว), "to be chaste" (lit. "to love and reserve one's body"), is an often-heard expression, especially in discussions about sex education and sexual behavior among youth. It reflects the normative values and expectations that Thai society has for women, and its invocation calls for women to exert restraint in their contact with the opposite sex, to refrain from gestures and verbal expressions that are obviously sexual, to make sure that men cannot sexually violate them, and to never enter into a relationship with someone else's partner. For a married woman, this ideal also implies being faithful and loving one's husband. According to Thai belief, a woman who is seen to be living according to the injunction *rak nuan sa-nguan tua*, "love and reserve your body," will be admired by both men and women, and she herself will feel that she is worthwhile and has honor that will be respected by men.[1]

Almost all of Thai literature reflects the long history of the importance given to *rak nuan sa-nguan tua*, from classical poems and epics such as *Khun Chang Khun Phaen*, the *Ramakien*, and *Inao*, to many contemporary novels. All consider *rak nuan sa-nguan tua* to be a measure of a woman's honor, and a criterion of being a *kunlasatri Thai* (กุลสตรีไทย), a "proper," "genteel," or "ladylike Thai woman," which every Thai woman is expected to be. Rachel Harrison has traced the persistence of conservative attitudes to female sexuality in both classical and modern Thai literature.[2]

It is noteworthy that while the Thai term for a "gentleman" or a "son of a noble or illustrious family," *kunlabut*, is not linked with ideas of sexual virtue, virginity or celibacy, the parallel term for a "gentlewoman" or "daughter of an illustrious family," *kunlasatri*, is intimately linked with ideas of *rak nuan sa-nguan tua*.

In ancient times, ladies in the royal court were brought up separately from men, and they had hardly any opportunity to meet members of the opposite sex. If a man touched a woman, even slightly, it was a big issue, since the woman could then be considered the man's wife. In the premodern period, the meaning of *rak nuan sa-nguan tua* may indeed have been literal. A woman had to "reserve her body" (*sa-nguan tua*) by not letting any man touch her. Later, due to foreign influences, the concept was linked to ideas of preserving virginity, *phrommajari* (พรหมจารี). Contemporary Thai society is now undergoing major changes, as gender- and sexuality-related values are continually influenced by the West, Japan, and other regions and countries. Clothing can now be more revealing, and greetings may involve hugging and touching. Women's increased role in public settings has resulted in more opportunities for interaction between women and men, and the issue of touching between a man and a woman has lost much of its importance. *Rak nuan sa-nguan tua* now tends to refer mostly to a woman maintaining her virginity before marriage. This is especially true for teenage girls who, in the eyes of broader society, should not engage in premarital sex. The activities of teenage girls are thus constantly under society's gaze.

Historians like Sujit Wongthes believe that the ideas associated with *kunlasatri* (being a virtuous woman), *rak nuan sa-nguan tua* (remaining chaste), *phrommajari* (virginity), and *phrommajan* (พรหมจรรย์) (celibacy) were spread through the Thai ruling class in the nineteenth century during the reign of King Rama IV (r. 1851–68), as they came in contact with the influence of Western, Victorian sexual values:

> Contrary to popular belief, female virginity (*phrommajari*) is a Western concept, not a Thai one. Powerful people today tend to say that the obligation for women to *rak nuan sa-nguan tua* and to be virginal is a true Thai tradition. However, it can be observed that in the *kuan khao thip* (กวนข้าวทิพย์) rice harvest festival, in which virginal women were required to officiate, they had to use girls under twelve years of age who had not yet menstruated, because people back then knew that around the time menstruation begins, at thirteen, children start to have sexual feelings. Hence, girls aged thirteen had a ceremony, called *berk phrommajan* (เบิก พรหมจรรย์), "opening the hymen" (from Chinese documents found in Cambodia), to mark the transition from being a child to a young lady. This was followed by *tham khwan* (ทำขวัญ), an encouragement ceremony, to prepare, in turn, for a *long khuang* (ลงข่วง) ceremony, which meant opening up an opportunity for youngsters to chat and get to know each other, leading to dating and sex if there was enough

mutual affection. But all this had to be under the control of the house tutelary spirits, and the elders in the house had to be in the know and ask for the spirits' forgiveness if sexual activity took place. The elders would then permit the young couple to live together without any harm being seen to be done. Subsequently if the couple could not get along together, they would break up.[3]

Many other terms are also used to teach, warn, or punish women in matters of sexual restraint. *Ot priao (wai) kin wan* (อดเปรี้ยว[ไว้]กินหวาน), "to abstain from the sour/sexy, to (later) eat sweets" (*priao* means both "to be sour" and "to be sexy"), and (*ya*) *ching suk korn ham* ([อย่า] ชิงสุกก่อนห่าม), "(don't) rush to ripeness before things are half-ripe," can be used for both men and women, but are usually used for only women, because Thai society assigns different values to men and women having sex. *Ot priao wai kin wan* means to refrain from something that is not good in order to gain something better later on, or to patiently wait for the reward ahead. In sexual matters it means refraining from having sex until an appropriate time, usually considered to be one's wedding day.[19] *Suk korn ham* means to do something prematurely, making a comparison with fruit that needs to ripen (*ham*) before it can be fully ripe (*suk*) enough to eat.[20] The expression is used to criticize inexperienced teenagers for starting to have sex too early.[6]

This double standard can be seen again in the usage of the terms *sia tua* (เสียตัว), "to lose one's body," and *dai sia* (ได้เสีย), "to gain, to lose," both of which mean "to have sex." *Sia tua* is usually only used with regard to women and means to lose one's virginity to a man and to end up as a his wife. It is an ancient term found in King U Thong's law on husbands and wives.[7] *Dai sia* is also an ancient expression that is still used. It connotes a mutual agreement to have sex between a woman and a man who are not married. The thing "gained" (*dai*) by the man is pleasure or sexual conquest and the thing "lost" (*sia*) by the woman is her virginal body.[8]

From "Rhinos" to "Golden Flowers": Labels that Disparage Non-Compliance with *Rak Nuan Sa-Nguan Tua*

Since *rak nuan sa-nguan tua* is used as a criterion of a woman's honor, women who do not follow this ideal are criticized and looked down upon. In slang, colloquial, and formal variations, the Thai language contains many terms for condemning women whose behavior and sexual expressions do not conform to the ideals of *rak nuan sa-nguan tua*. These expressions range from quite soft ones to the truly coarse. Many of the terms in the following list are also used by, and about, sexually promiscuous *gays* and *kathoeys*. However, in these cases they may be playful, ironic compliments, rather than derogatory terms:

datjarit (ดัดจริต): v. to be insincere, to overact or be affected in one's actions or speech, also often used of effeminate *gays* and *kathoeys*.[9]

dae-dae (แดะแด๋ or แด๊ะแด๋): v. (1) to overact, to be insincere or affected, as in "He's a real man (*phu-chai thae thae*) but can act *dae-dae* like a real *kathoey*;" (2) to be animated, move around in a cute way, as in "This dog's so *dae-dae*, trying to please its owner so much;" (3) to parade around, as in "Each day, she does no work, and just goes around *dae-dae* all the time."[10]

ran (ร่าน): v. (1) to want sexually, to lust after (usually used in a sexual sense); (2) to rush or hurry.[11]

raet (แรด): literally means a "rhinoceros." Some informants have speculated that its use as a word of abuse for women, *gays*, and *kathoeys* refers to the female rhinoceros' strong sex drive in the mating season, during which she might even butt the male rhino to death. As a slang word, it has several definitions:

(coll.) v. *datjarit*, see above.[12]
    v. to behave in a shamefully dissolute and flirtatious way, as in "Girls these days are so *raet*, having boyfriends from such an early age." This same category also includes the expression *sip-et ror. dor.* (11 ร.ด.) and *hok-sip hok ror. dor.* (66 ร.ด.), which are both indirect references to *raet*, as in "*Sip-et ror. dor.* like this . . . watch out or you might not get the diapers in time [for the new baby]." These expressions come from the fact that in Thai the numbers eleven (*sip-et*) and sixty-six (*hok-sip hok*) look similar to the Thai vowel symbol แ, which is the first written element of *raet*, while *ror. dor.* is the spelling of the two consonants in this word. *Raet ngiap* (แรดเงียบ), "to *raet* quietly," and *raet lop nai* (แรดหลบใน), "to *raet* covertly," refer to similar, but more discreet behavior, as in "This superstar is *raet ngiap*, pretending to be ever so proper, but secretly changes partners at whim."[13]

Words with a meaning similar to *raet* or *datjarit* are also found in regional Thai dialects. *Haen* (แอ่น) and *salit* (สะหลิด) are found in Northern Thai. *Haet* (แฮด) and *hee khiao* (หีเคียว), "sickle cunt," are used in Northeastern Thai. In both Northern and Northeastern Thai, the Central Thai "r" is often pronounced as "h," hence *raet* is pronounced *haet*. In Southern Thai *or ror* (อ้อร้อ) has a similar meaning.[14]

The words *phaetsaya* (แพศยา) and (*ee*) *dork thorng* ([อี]ดอกทอง) are ancient terms that have been found in law texts and literature since the Ayutthayan era, and are defined in the *Dictionary of the Royal Institute* as:

phaetsaya: n. a woman seeking livelihood from prostitution; an evil, mean, promiscuous woman (S. *ves'ya*; P. *vesiya*).[15]

dork thorng: n. a woman of easy virtue, slut (a term of abuse).[16]

Various explanations have been offered for the origins of the expression *dork thorng*. Some view it is a corruption of the Teochew Chinese *lok thong* (หลกทั่ง), which means "as red as hot iron," and likewise refers to sexually insatiable women. Others think *dork thorng* refers to the reddish flowers of *Butea monosperma Kuntze*, which is colloquially called *ton dork thorng* (ต้นดอกทอง), "golden flower tree." Along with brothels, these trees used to be common around the old red-light district in the Sampeng market area of Bangkok, and men would say they had visited "golden flower houses." This is said to be a possible basis for the link between *dork thorng* and female sex workers. *Dork thorng* has also been linked to the name of a pungent herb that supposedly makes anyone sniffing it sexually aroused. *Dork thorng* might also be a word play on *dorng thork* (ดองถอก), a slang reference to the male sexual organ, denoting a "penis" (*dorng*) that has the "foreskin pulled back" (*thork*). Yet another explanation is that the word refers to patterns on the skin of the *tua ngern tua thorng* (ตัวเงินตัวทอง), "monitor lizard," which Thai people detest, and the animal's name may have been introduced as a word of abuse for women who behave badly. Finally, *dork thorng* also refers to reddish flowers in general, and red (being the color of blood) is also the color of *Kali*, the Hindu goddess that supposedly has a liking for orgiastic tantric ceremonies of worship.[17] Kali is a symbol of promiscuity, and the name Kali (กาลี) might be the original form of yet another word of abuse for sexually promiscuous women, *krari* (กระหรี่), or "whore."[18]

While women who have sex with many men are coarsely condemned as *dork thorng*, men who behave similarly not only avoid condemnation, but are even made objects of admiration with expressions like *chai chatri* (ชายชาตรี), "he-man." As one commentator observes: "Conversely, let men consider this in regard to a woman's promiscuity, and it will become a scandal for her: *ee nang kaki,* or more brutally, *ee dork thorng*! ("damn slut!" "damn whore!"). An example might be a married couple who live together and have a son or a daughter—if the husband has a minor wife, parts of society can accept that; but if the wife does the same with a man, society will not accept it or let it happen."[19]

A Sexual Ideology that Oppresses Women and Leads to Sexual Health Problems

Thai society has high expectations for women and strictly controls their behavior, including sexual behavior. This can be seen from the number of terms available to attack a woman's sense of being a good woman, as society defines it. Of these, *rak nuan sa-nguan tua* is perhaps the harshest, as a term used to control women's sexualities; as an idiom, it is encountered in every societal context: homes, educational institutions, the medical establishment, religion, and the mass media. Whenever news emerges about young people having sex, especially when a public festival (during which young people might have sex)[32] is approaching, the media works with state and private organizations to intensify their campaigns among youth to promote the ideology of *rak nuan sa-nguan tua*. An example of one such campaign is a *rak nuan sa-nguan tua* club founded by a well-known female senator. This club campaigns in schools to make young people (who are viewed as not abiding by the dictates of *rak nuan sa-nguan tua*) embrace this value and behave according to presumed Thai traditions. Other examples include:

- A campaign with stickers on Bangkok buses urging teenagers to "take care of their hearts and bodies, both men and women, to preserve [Thai] culture" (*raksa jai raksa kai thang ying chai rak watthanatham*).
- The "10 No's" (*khatha 10 ya*) campaign by the Royal Thai Police targeting young women.[20]
- Campaigning, training courses, and a youth manual for *rak nuan sa-nguan tua* by the Council of the Women of Thailand, aimed at instilling the value of *rak nuan sa-nguan tua* and promoting health among young women.[21]

In Thai society, it is hoped that by preventing women and girls from having sex at a young age and encouraging them to abide by the dictates of *rak nuan sa-nguan tua* they will be protected from sex-related problems. Society hopes this will eliminate unwanted pregnancies, abortions, HIV infection, and sexual violence. However, women and girls are likely to continue to encounter these problems, as they have in the past, as a consequence of the mainstream gender and sexuality value system that reproduces patriarchal power. Perhaps no extent of campaigning for *rak nuan sa-nguan tua* will reduce these problems because the ideology of *rak nuan sa-nguan tua* perpetuates a system of control over women's sexualities. Implicit in this system of control is the misguided belief that "good women" have no desire to learn about sexual matters or express their views on such matters. The result is that women of all ages are prevented from learning about safe sex and sexual pleasure and are left unprepared to deal with sexual health problems. Women are made to feel embarrassed about exchanging sex-related ideas, learning about their bodies, communicating with their partners about safe sex and mutual sexual pleasure, seeing sexual health service providers, and speaking with such health providers directly enough to enable them to provide a correct diagnosis for whatever their health problems may be.

Sexuality Studies: Issues of Sex, Lifestyle, and Sexual Rights

In Thai society sexual matters are considered sensitive and private matters that should be hidden. *Rak nuan sa-nguan tua* has been the main framework for state attempts to reduce sexual problems and prevent the spread of HIV infection among young women. Various institutions continue to tell youth that since they are the nation's future, they are not yet of an appropriate age to have anything to do with sexual matters. These ideas match Victorian sexual ideology, a part of Thai cultural heritage since the era of King Chulalongkorn, Rama V (r. 1868–1910).[22]

Rak nuan sa-nguan tua tends to be used in conjunction with the formal expression *kan mi phet-samphan korn wai an khuan* (การมีเพศสัมพันธ์ก่อนวัยอันควร), "having sex before an appropriate age," which can be understood in various ways. From a sociocultural point of view, children and youth (those still studying at school or university) can be seen as being too young for sex due to their not having the maturity and responsibility to deal with its consequences.[23] Alternatively, from an anatomical point of view, this expression suggests that having sex at an age at which the sexual organs are still not fully mature may, in turn, lead to physical damage to the organs or to transmission of STDs. However, most people tend to think of the former explanation, which is linked to *rak nuan sa-nguan tua,* when speaking of having sex "too early."

Traditionally, sex educators in Thailand have placed a great deal of emphasis on preventing youth from having sex and teaching them *rak nuan sa-nguan tua.* Seeing sexual matters as merely anatomical differences between men and women, or teaching youth to control their sexual feelings by engaging in other activities, such as sports, cannot provide answers to the questions that young people may have about sex, and are also at odds with the sexual content of various modern media that youth can easily access.

To facilitate analytical, critical abilities among children and youth, sex education should focus on language and its role in the perpetuation of sexual ideologies. It should also analyze Thai sexual traditions and cultures in order to understand the gender order they conceal, and which controls masculinity and femininity as well as all sexualities. Sex education should be aimed at increasing children's and young people's ability to think about sexual phenomena within modern society and to understand that sex and sexuality are not "problems" (*panha*), but rather are a part of being human, a mixture of culture and sociocultural meanings, feelings, preferences, choices, attitudes, and selfhoods. Everyone should consider sexual rights as basic human rights: the right to choose one's gender/sex (*phet*), gender/sexual expression, and sexuality. Learning about sexual matters should lead to deeper analysis of the conservative socializing processes and the instilling of gender and sexuality-related beliefs that leave women without the knowledge and ability to make independent decisions as to how to lead their sexual lives.

Rak nuan sa-nguan tua reflects the sexual oppression of women in Thai society. It is the moralistic slogan of campaigns driven by the ideology of "sex within marriage/adult sex=legitimate sex." Its widespread use in such campaigns reflects the expectations and gender roles that direct ideologies controlling youth and female sexualities, while failing to analyze the sociocultural context that, in fact, pushes children and youth to have sex while still studying. Power relations are an important variable when children and women negotiate sex. *Rak nuan sa-nguan tua* seems to go against the flows of the shifting currents of sexual values and beliefs in Thai society today. It does not match the changes occurring in Thai society and Thai youth sexual cultures under the influences of globalization and consumerism. Campaigning to promote this value not only fails to provide youth with analytic tools to deal with sexual matters (and thereby liberate themselves from the confines of an unequal gender order that constitutes a risk factor for sexual ill-being), it also fails to consider the sexual human rights of young people that would guarantee them the right to have safe, consensual sex of the kind they themselves choose to have.

3 *KHUN PHAEN* (ขุนแผน): A WOMANIZER

Sulaiporn Chonwilai

Khun Phaen: The Archetypal Thai Womanizer

Khun Phaen (alternate transcriptions include *Kunpan, Khunpan,* and *Kun Pan*) (ขุนแผน) is the name of a lead male character in the classical Thai literary work *Khun Chang Khun Phaen,* which is based on an orally transmitted story from the Ayutthaya period (fourteenth to eighteenth centuries CE) that was then collated and written down in the early Rattanakosin era. This highly popular classic represents a love triangle connecting Khun Phaen and Khun Chang— *khun* being the lowest rank of ancient Thai nobility—and Lady Wanthorng.[1] Given *Khun Phaen*'s reputation for his skill both in battle and with women, it is unsurprising that his name in Thai folklore has become a synonym for *jao chu* (เจ้าชู้), "womanizer."

   Khun Phaen is by no means the only womanizing lead male character in classical Thai literature. Lead male characters in other works such as *Phra Aphai Mani* and *Inao* all have several wives. Premodern Thai society considered the number of wives a man had a measure of his charisma and power. Being a womanizer is thus one of the qualifications for a true Thai lead male character. However, *Khun Phaen* differs from other womanizing lead male characters in classical literature in that he is a commoner, not of royal stock, and prey to everyday human emotions like love, greed, anger, and infatuation. He has come to be seen as something of an archetype of the ideal Thai man, represented as a strong leader who is clever, loyal to his benefactors, and skilled both in love and war. His "charm" (*saneh*) is made evident by his having five wives.

   However, younger people who have not grown up imbibing the Thai literary classics, and city dwellers whose lifestyles do not involve the old traditions that remain strong in the countryside, seem to consider the term *Khun Phaen* outdated. Other terms such as *playboy* (เพลย์บอย), *Casanova* (คาสซาโนว่า), *phraya the khrua* (พระยาเทครัว), and *seua phu-ying* (เสือผู้หญิง) also refer to womanizers, with varying connotations.

Playboy, for example, is an English loanword that in its Thai usage denotes a "rich man who does not work and devotes himself to a life of pleasure without commitments or responsibilities."[2] Originally, the definition of *playboy* in English was not limited to womanizing behavior, but the word came to be used almost exclusively in that sense due to the influence of *Playboy* magazine, America's most famous men's magazine, which has been published since 1953. During the Vietnam War, there were large numbers of American soldiers in Thailand, which increased Thai society's familiarity both with the magazine and American culture more generally. Narong Chanruang, author of the Mit Nam-meuk ("Ink Friend") newspaper column, wrote that in that era nighttime entertainment venue owners were keen to use the term *playboy* in their establishments' names— whether clubs, bars, hotels, or motels—and that Thai men of all ages, social classes, and occupations aspired to be *playboys*. Rong Wongsawan, a veteran writer whose works mostly reflect the feelings and sexual lives of men, once said in an interview that being a *playboy* is not easy:

> Even if you're a millionaire, if you don't have any other abilities besides buying women or using a twenty-carat diamond ring to dry your wife's tears, you're not a *playboy*. A *playboy* has to be the fox and the tiger of the concrete jungle. He has to be skilled, have good taste, as well as both compassion and brutality within him. I think there are no more than a few *playboys* in Thailand.[3]

Today, the term *playboy* is well-known and often used by the media when referring to male superstars or famous people who are known womanizers.

The same is true for *Casanova,* another foreign term introduced to Thailand. Casanova was an Italian adventurer and writer who lived from 1725 to 1798 and whose story as a great lover and philanderer has been presented (sometimes twisted) in numerous books and motion pictures.[4] It is thought he had sex with more than two hundred women belonging to all social classes living all over Europe. It is little wonder, then, that his name has become a synonym for a womanizer. It is hard to ascertain when the name *Casanova* reached Thailand, but it is thought that the media and educated, upper-class people played a major role in making it a well-known term. To be called *Casanova,* one needs to be a young man of good background, well-known, and reportedly involved with

44

numerous women. The words *playboy* and *Casanova* reflect the influence of Western languages and cultures on Thai society. The terms also reflect the social class and context of the communicators using them, although both are now well-known in Thai.

In contrast, *phraya the khrua* is an old Thai term that refers to a womanizing man who gets all the women in the same family or clan as his wives. Khun Wichitmatra explained that *the khrua* means a "married man with a house, who gathers all the sisters or other relatives of his wife, as well as all the servant women in the house, as his wives."[5] This expression, combined with *phraya,* a Thai nobility rank, is probably linked to cases of such behavior by persons with that rank in the past, because they had plenty of servants (or slaves) in their houses. Khun Wichitmatra concluded that money and power were necessary to be a *phraya the khrua,* but the *phraya* rank itself was not. The term is now used only rarely, because societal changes have given women more freedom and decreased their economic dependence on men. Married couples tend to move out of their parents' house, and the law now allows men only one wife (although many Thai men maintain mistresses or "minor wives," *mia noi*). These changes have made it rare for a man to have several wives who are sisters or otherwise related to each other. News of young men marrying two sisters now usually involves the husband sexually harassing or even raping another woman in the wife's family.

Similar to the term "lady-killer" in English, *seua phu-ying* is an expression that refers to a man skilled in wooing women (to appease his endless sexual appetite), and compares him with a tiger preying on its victim. The tiger, having finished up one victim, goes to look for the next one. Used between men, the term reflects a show of admiration for womanizing abilities, for having power over women, and not being bound by them. For women, the term implies an untrustworthy man who views women exclusively as sex objects. In modern Thai society, although womanizing behavior is still held in high esteem, values related to love, mutual faithfulness, and monogamous relationships are now very important in whether or not a man is considered a good partner or husband. While it is considered normal for men to have womanizing habits, a wife or a partner who would accept the behavior of a *seua phu-ying* would be hard to come by.

Jao Chu: A Sexual Freedom Denied to Women

The *Dictionary of the Royal Institute* defines the term *jao chu* as "a person who engages in adultery."[6] While it can be used for both men and women, Thai society judges the value of male and female *jao chu* very differently. Historical variations of this term include:

jao chu kai jae (เจ้าชู้ไก่แจ้): a man who intentionally exhibits *jao chu* behavior toward women, like a bantam rooster, or *kai jae,* that struts about to show its interest in hens.

jao chu yak (เจ้าชู้ยักษ์): a "giant *jao chu,*" a man who courts women inconsiderately or outright violently, like giants (*yak*) in Thai classical drama.

jao chu pratu din (เจ้าชู้ประตูดิน): *pratu din* is the name for an inner gate on the Tha Tien side of the Grand Palace in Bangkok. In the past, men were not allowed to enter the palace through this gate, and those with a taste for palace ladies, called *jao chu pratu din,* had to congregate outside this gate to court such ladies as they went in and out of the palace.

The above expressions were used for men only. While they may appear to convey negative implications, they, in fact, only describe, rather than condemn, different types of *jao chu,* implicitly accepting that being a man (*phu-chai*) and being a *jao chu* belong together.

Thai society permits men, not women, to be *jao chu.* A woman is still expected to behave like a *kunlasatri* (กุลสตรี), a "ladylike woman," to be chaste or *rak nuan sa-nguan tua,* not to have sex with men before marriage and, when married, *rak diao jai diao* (รักเดียวใจเดียว), "to love only one [person] and be faithful" to him. Yet, a woman does not even need to have sex with anyone to be stigmatized by society as not being a "good woman." This can also happen if she lapses in watching her manners or sexual expressions when men are present. The Thai language has many words for condemning, or even verbally abusing, women who are seen as *jao chu* or as engaging in sexual behavior that does not match societal expectations. Such terms include *ran* (ร่าน), *raet* (แรด), *phaetsaya* (แพศยา), *dork thorng* (ดอกทอง), and *samsorn* (สำส่อน), all of which refer to promiscuity in some way (see chapter 2).

While the names *Khun Phaen* and *Casanova* reveal some admiration for the men they are used to refer to, no woman would like to be compared with

Wanthorng, Mora (โมรา), or Kaki (กากี), all names of women from classical literature who had several husbands. These figures can be found in three Thai literary works, *Khun Chang Khun Phaen, Chantakorop,* and *Kaki.* The authors of these works, presumably all men,[7] show that in addition to verbal abuse, women also receive harsh punishments for violating society's sexual standards. Wanthorng is sentenced to death, Mora is cursed and transformed into a gibbon, and Kaki is left on a raft in the middle of the ocean. Their names have become symbols of so-called "bad women" (*phu-ying chua*) worthy of severe criticism, and their names are also found in expressions used to condemn women, such as *Wanthorng sorng jai* (วันทองสองใจ), "two-hearted (i.e., unfaithful) Wanthorng," and *pen yang nang Kaki* (เป็นอย่างนางกากี), "to be like Lady Kaki."

Thai women and men are now more equal than before, but Thai women still cannot escape the expectation that they should follow old societal mores in sexual matters. However, women's increased educational opportunities and independence, together with the influence of media in our age of borderless communication, have made women more receptive to liberal ideas about sexual matters. This, in turn, has made women dare to challenge and negotiate sexual matters more than they did previously. Today, women recognize that they have the right to lead their sexual lives as they wish, just as men do. Unmarried women may now have more choice in terms of whom to date or in terms of changing their partners than they did in the past. This can be seen in the media portrayal of several female superstars who are known to have changed their partners many times, and are referred to as *Casanovi,* or female *Casanovas.* Those thus represented, however, are not usually particularly happy about this portrayal because they do not wish to be judged as having gender/sexual (*phet*) expressions that are outside the societal frame in such matters.

Attitudes about being a *jao chu* are related to the unequal value assigned to different genders (*phet*) in Thai society. This not only affects the sexual relations and lives of heterosexuals, but also the sexualities of homosexual people, which also reflect the societal binary division of genders. For example, most *toms,* or masculine lesbians (see chapter 12), reject the femininity that society expects of them, and instead use the value gained by being linked with masculinity—part of which is being considered to be a *jao chu*—to construct their identities. *Gays,* on the other hand, have even greater freedom of sexual expression by virtue of being male, but the more they make use of this male privilege of sexual freedom in their lives, the more prejudice they encounter regarding their sexual behavior. Because *gays, toms, dees,* and homosexuals of other sexual identities have sex for pleasure and not for procreation, society sees their relationships as short-lived and promiscuous, involving the risk of being infected with STDs and spreading these diseases further into society. Hence, it can be said that the value of being a *jao chu* is judged using unequal standards for people of different gender and sexual identities.

From "Unfaithful Women" (*phu-ying lai jai*) to *Jao Chu* Men: Health Consequences of the Language of Inequality

Society allows men to be *jao chu*—explaining this by referencing their supposedly stronger sexual needs and by citing various scientific and psychological theories. By contrast, it exerts strict control on women's sexual behavior through expressions like *rak nuan sa-nguan tua* and *rak diao jai diao*, which leads to sexual inequality and various health consequences. For example, it is considered normal and a matter of gaining life experience that men have premarital sex, but women doing the same are considered unworthy. Few women dare to ask their husbands to use condoms, even if they know their husband is having sex with others, because decision-making power on the issue lies with the husband. Women have to endure flirtation (e.g., words, gazes, and actions of men) that could be considered sexual harassment, but which is ignored by a society that views these things as normal behavior for men.

Competition among men to gain sexual experiences with women, as well as their desire to gain acceptance from their friends, can lead to rape and sexual violence. Men's sexual jealousy may lead to physical, psychological, and sexual violence against their lovers or wives.

In same-sex couples, when one party behaves in a *jao chu* manner, relationship problems similar to those found in heterosexual couples emerge. Interestingly, the use of the expression "being a *jao chu*" among people of different sexual identities reflects gender role divisions between masculine and feminine parties in such relationships. The terms *playboy, Khun Phaen,* and *Casanova* tend to be used for *toms* who also are *jao chu,* but not for *gays* or men who love men (*chai rak chai*), who more commonly tend to be labeled *samsorn* or "promiscuous." This use of a term with feminine connotations to refer to *gays* who have multiple sexual partners reflects the societal perception of them as men who reject their masculinity by choosing to have sex with other men.

The different values assigned to different genders (both among heterosexuals and those involved in same-sex relationships) reflected in the *jao chu* concept, as well as the power given by society to men to control both their own and women's sex lives, pose risks for various sexual health problems. These risks include the possibility of sexual violence and harassment against women, women being forced to have sex to satisfy men's needs, unwanted pregnancies, STDs and HIV/AIDS as well as prejudice and discrimination in the provision of sexual health services for people who have sex with members of their own sex. While specific sexual health services have been set up for men who love men, these services still perpetuate the prejudice that these men have to be monitored, because they are perceived to be a source of the spread of HIV infection, as a result of presumed promiscuous behavior. On the other hand, there is a dearth of information on the sexual health of women who have sex with women, and a lack of attention to their sexual behaviors, which leads to their exclusion from sexual health services, whether they engage in risky sexual behavior or not.

All of this, from *Khun Phaen* to the "two-hearted" *Wanthorng*, reflects perspectives on men and women in Thai society, as well as their unequal social standing. As long as this sexual inequality, reflected in the connotations of the terms discussed above, remains invisible, people of all gender and sexual identities will continue to face risks and suffer the relationship problems linked to it.

4 *KHEUN KHAN* (ขึ้นคาน): TO BE A SPINSTER

Sulaiporn Chonwilai

A (Not So) Ancient Thai Idiom

kheun khan (ขึ้นคาน), "to go into dry dock," is an old Thai expression that remains in use today. Literally it means lifting a boat onto dry land and putting it up on wooden beams, that is, putting it into dry dock for repairs. Metaphorically, it refers to a "woman who is no longer young but remains unmarried."[1] A boat is lifted up onto dry land for repair because it is old, in bad shape, and unusable, and the expression applies these meanings to women. Kanjanakhaphan defines the meaning of *kheun khan* as follows:

> *kheun khan*: all alone—usually used of women who have been abandoned by their husbands, and so have to live alone; of young women who do not have an opportunity to find a suitable partner, for example, due to their high social status or affluence, no man dares to approach them, and they have to stay alone; or of older unmarried women who [due to their age] do not think of looking for a partner or whom no man seeks.[2]

In the past, *kheun khan* had two meanings, denoting either a divorced woman or a single woman, but nowadays it is primarily used only for the latter. Divorced women now tend to be called *mae mai* (แม่ม่าย), a "widow." Some expressions that denote a single woman have already fallen out of use, while others remain in use in some regions of the country. For example, the *Dictionary of the Royal Institute* defines *sao theun theuk* or *sao theum theuk* (สาวทึนทึก/สาวทึมทึก) as "an elder, still unmarried woman, or a *sao theua* (สาวเทื้อ)."[3] The expression *theum theuk* refers to almost ripe coconuts, which are called *maphrao theum theuk* (มะพร้าว

ทึมทึก). In the expression *sao theua,* the word *sao* refers to *sao kae,* "woman," and the word *theua* refers to *theun theuk,* meaning "not active."[4] Internet searches suggest that *sao theua* is an old term because it is used in the Thai translation of the Theravada Buddhist scriptures, the *Tripitaka* (*Vinayapitaka,* vol. 2, verse 181), in relation to the regulations governing monks' behavior: "Women who are prostitutes, widows, *sao theua,* or nuns, as well as *kathoeys,* should not visit monks unnecessarily, or at an inappropriate time."[5] *Sao khern* (สาวเคิ้น) is a Northern Thai term that refers to unmarried women. *Khern* means "to be left or leftover," as in "A vendor goes to the market to sell goods, but as not all of the goods are sold, some are *khern.*"[6] *Sao kae* (สาวแก่), an "old maid," or in Northern Thai, *sao thao* (สาวเฒ่า/ สาวเถ้า), are yet more expressions for women who remain unmarried into old age.

All of these terms are derogatory and used exclusively or mostly about women. Thai society expects both men and women to have a partner (of the opposite sex) and to get married at an appropriate age. For example, in Northern Thailand, if a young woman or man has not found a partner by the age of thirty, and does not have a family, it is considered embarrassing. It is thought that there will not be anyone for him or her anymore, and he or she is called *bao khern* (บ่าวเคิ้น) or *bao thao* (บ่าวเถ้า), an "old bachelor," or *sao khern* or *sao thao,* an "old maid."[7]

However, women typically face more pressure than men to marry. Women are expected to marry a man who is the same age or older than themselves, while the opposite is true for men. Women who get married when they are over thirty years old are considered slow in getting married, and yet it is considered normal for men to get married when they are over thirty. Society sees unmarried, single women as women who have not been chosen, whom nobody wants, and who are "unsaleable" on the marriage market. Single men are not seen in the same light. Rather, they are seen as men who are concerned about maintaining their freedom, because society permits pre-marital sex for men, viewing it as unproblematic or even a matter of course. The more a single man socializes with women, the more charismatic (or the more of a womanizer) he is considered to be. However, it is also generally held that women have to be chaste (see chapter 2) until marriage, due to the fact that it is the norm for the man to be the party proposing marriage. Present-day Thai society still does not tolerate premarital or extramarital sex for women. Yet women who remain single past a certain age are considered abnormal for not having been courted by a man, which causes many women to get married even if they are still uncertain about their readiness for life as part of a couple, thinking they better get married before it is too late.

From An Ordinary Dry Dock to "Miss Golden Dry Dock"

Kheun khan is widely used for women of all social classes, regardless of their wealth, educational status, or religion. Increasingly, many Thai women *kheun khan*, or remain unmarried, whether intentionally or not, as a result of societal changes that have granted them greater economic self-reliance through educational and employment opportunities. They now see marriage as a right or a choice rather than an economic or societal necessity.

In the past, women did not have educational opportunities, and for both economic and societal reasons could not live independently. For rural women, marriage not only meant perpetuating their families, but also increasing the labor force in the house, because men were expected to help their wives make a living and manage the financial assets of the family. For upper-class women, marriage meant the possibility of further upward mobility and gaining a protector. Upper-class women had hardly any opportunities to experience life outside of their homes, and for them marriage tended to be a matter of their parents finding a man whom they considered suitable for their daughter. A woman was simply a transferable asset for the parents and for the husband. This, coupled with the legal and social opportunities that in the past gave Thai men the right to have several wives, made it almost impossible for a woman to remain single past what was considered marrying age. Hence, it is not strange that Thai people used to perceive women "in dry dock" negatively, and as being abnormal in some respect for not having had any man ask for their hand.

Surveys among Bangkok women conducted between 1960 and 2000 by the Institute for Population and Social Research at Mahidol University confirm that the proportion of women staying unmarried has steadily increased, reflecting societal changes.[8] Values and attitudes towards having a partner and marriage have also changed. Marrying for love is now valued more than marrying for economic necessity, and only monogamy is now accepted. However, Thai society still holds to a family ideology based on heterosexuality and patriarchy. Thus, pressure remains on Thai women to marry and to have a family, which means gaining a protector and children to continue the family line, as well as fulfilling the duties of a good wife and mother, which in turn fulfill the family's and society's expectation that the woman be *kunlasatri* (กุลสตรี), a "proper" or "genteel" lady. These pressures are reflected in the following postings to web board discussions:

Today, I went to a relative's wedding. Yet another one getting married. And I felt awkward, because of all the questions as to when I will marry, if I'd like them to look for a fiancé for me, something like this. Ever since I got my bachelors degree, all my relatives keep asking, my grandparents, my uncle, my aunt, everyone . . . [9]

I'm almost thirty now; we've been a couple for about eight years. I also get asked when I'll get married, and so we did get engaged last year. But it's still the same old "When will you get married?" I guess it'll be like this until I finally do. And it's not just me who gets asked. My mum also gets asked about me, and it stresses her, because her daughter's this old already. It's serious enough for me not to feel like going back home or meeting anyone there. I told my mum to tell them that we've already separated, to put an end to those questions. The reason I haven't gotten married yet is that I don't feel ready . . . [due to lack of economic] security, and what's more, my partner's folks saw an astrologer, and the astrologer said he must marry at thirty-three, for us to be able to stay together forever. Wow! Not having anyone to marry is torture, but so is having someone and having to wait. I've worried to the point I can't be bothered anymore. I'll let it go by its own nature. [51]

The anxieties of a woman afraid of *kheun khan*, or "staying in dry dock," waiting for a man to ask for her hand, are expressed in a song by female singer Siriphorn Amphaiphong:

They call me a "golden dry dock angel" . . . sad whenever I hear it.
Face getting older, body not so slender, but still I'm a "Miss."
Wrinkles in the mirror as I smile at it, I dream of the giver of a promise
Who always told me to wait, and my heart still dares to wait.
To other men I said no. I kept my red cheeks. I waited for you, you know?
Mum and Dad said "He's cheating on you." I count the years, tears running . . . [11]

The expression *kheun khan* comes with the perception that a woman who is over thirty and still chooses to be without a partner must be somehow abnormal. People either think that she is not smart or talented or else she is too much into religion, which men find unattractive. Or perhaps people think her personality is too unstable, or her habits are too strange for anyone to take a look at her. Or worse still, maybe they think she hates men and likes women instead. What women can do to deal with this type of prejudice against single women is to create new meanings for the term *kheun khan* and to spread positive perspectives about single women. One example of this is contending that although one has "gone into dry dock," the docks in question are *khan thorng* (คานทอง), "golden docks," a reference to the status or wealth that make men meaningless as economic providers and in terms of social status. A humorous legend on the origins of the expression "golden docks," *khan thorng,* is often cited on the Internet:

> A long, long time ago, there was a rich man, who announced that whoever wants to marry his daughter, will have to bring a million *chang* [1 *chang* equals 1.2 kg] of gold as the bride price. A poor man, who was the lover of the rich man's daughter, decided to go far, far away to dig for gold, in order to be able to ask for the rich man's daughter's hand. Thirty years passed, and the poor man brought in all the gold the rich man had requested. But the young woman had become an old spinster, and the man could not take it that she had lost her beauty. He lost his senses and died, leaving all the gold to the rich man's daughter. And so the rich man's daughter took all the gold to build a golden dock to sit on and listen to music to her heart's content, and then left it for future generations as a reminder of her story.[12]

Khan thorng became a hot topic when the mass media reported on the first *Miss Khan Thorng* (มิสคานทอง), or "Miss Golden Docks," competition in 2003. The competition was held to select a beautiful single woman age thirty or over as *Miss Khan Thorng,* who would then participate in various kinds of charity work. Important objectives of the competition included (i) reminding women of their value, and the fact that even without a partner they can live their lives happily, (ii) challenging negative societal perceptions related to *kheun khan,* and (iii) respecting the right of women to make decisions regarding their own lives, including the decision to have a partner only when they themselves are ready, without fear that they will be left in "dry dock" (*kheun khan*) or be seen as different from others.[13] Thephatsadin Na Ayutthaya, the first winner of the competition explained that:

> Last year, quite a lot of men came to see the competition. And many of them were surprised, as they had thought single women had to be old, not beautiful, something like [the TV soap opera character] Mean Teacher Wai, but when they saw it . . . oh, it wasn't like that.[14]

Although the *Miss Khan Thorng* competition was an attempt to change societal attitudes towards single women aged thirty and over, it still gave primary emphasis to the contestants' appearance. What this reflects is that single women have to compensate for not having a partner by becoming exceptional in some other respect, such as by looking younger than their age or by having educational or professional achievements. A professional title, like "Dr.," can replace the personal title "Miss," which becomes awkward as one gets older. Failing this, single women may face malicious gossip. All of this creates pressure on women.

Popular expansions of *khan thorng* include *khan thorng niwet* (คานทองนิเวศน์), *chomrom khan thorng* (ชมรมคานทอง), and *samakhom khan thorng* (สมาคมคานทอง), which all refer to an idealized community of older unmarried women that provides them with friends similar to themselves, a chance for mutual reliance and support, and an opportunity to live their lives happily. These concepts are also reminders of the meaninglessness of values that pressure women to have a partner, as Sui Oe explains:

This expression *kheun khan* is outdated for unmarried women in our present-day society. It sounds oppressive and pitiable, like when a woman is not married nobody wants her. But really, they're people who have chosen their kind of happiness . . . Yes! They're not married, but they're a good daughter, a good person, known for their devotion to society . . . They can also be considered complete human beings. There are many kinds of single people in our country. They've got their reasons . . . Making the value judgment that a woman is better because she's got a partner is not right . . . the idiom the "association of golden docks" (*samakhom khan thorng*) doesn't scare women . . . They're traveling, they've got money in the bank, and lots of projects for the benefit of society.[15]

Overlooked Issues of Women in Dry Dock

Older single women especially tend to be seen as being on the prowl to catch an inexperienced young man or as having to marry the first possible man as their last resort. Women who stay in dry dock (*kheun khan*) may also be perceived as being frigid or homosexual. Even if such allegations are not meant seriously, they reflect control over women's sexualities. All women are expected to follow the model of monogamous, heterosexual marriage. Whether single or not, whether past the so-called marrying age or not, unlike men, Thai women are not given the right to have premarital or extramarital sex. Those who change their sex partners often are especially not accepted by society. A clear example of this patriarchal control of women was a Thai law that forced women to change their personal title from *nang sao* (นางสาว), "Miss," to *nang* (นาง), "Mrs.," upon marriage, while men continued to use the title *nai* (นาย), "Mr.," regardless of their marital status. This was the equivalent of letting everyone know a woman's marital status without giving her the right to choose when to disclose it, even though it is a matter of personal privacy. The Thai Personal Titles Act was recently changed. Now, its fifth article permits married women to choose whether to use *nang sao*, "Miss," or *nang*, "Mrs.," as their title, and the sixth article of the revised law gives the same right to divorced women. However, the related attempt to allow post-operative male-to-female transsexuals (aged fifteen and over and in possession of a doctor's certificate as proof of transsexual status) the legal right to choose their personal title as "Miss" rather "Mr." met with criticism and was rejected.

The only respect in which "dry-dock women" (*kheun khan*) are viewed positively is that they are considered as better off than homosexual women, and perhaps better off than *mai* (widows or divorcees), because at least they are seen as virginal and as still having some opportunities for marriage, more so than women who love women. The number of women who have a female partner, but publicly state they are single to cover up loving the same sex, may partially explain an apparent rise in the proportion of single women in society today.

The societal perception that women who are already in "dry dock" (*kheun khan*) will not have had sex (with either men or women) can affect these women's sexual health. Those who indeed have never had sex may neglect their sexual health—due to the mistaken belief that, never having had sex, their sexual organs cannot have any health problems—whereas those who have had sex may not dare to reveal their experiences to a doctor due to societal expectations. Both these situations may affect making a correct diagnosis or the provision of treatment.

The values and ideas reflected in the use of the expression *kheun khan* show that Thai society expects both men and women of a certain age to get married and to produce offspring, but single men and women are each seen in a different light. There are no words or expressions for ridiculing single men in Thai. In contrast, as much as women try to improve their status or to reclaim the expression *kheun khan,* the attitudes and values of patriarchal society still control them, exposing them to stress, pressure, and various other mental and physical health consequences, all mediated through the discursive power of this idiom.

5 *SIN SORT* (สินสอด): BRIDE PRICE

Sulaiporn Chonwilai

The Bride (Candidate)'s Value and Breast Milk Fee

Sin sort (สินสอด) is generally understood as either a bride price, which is the property that a man gives to a woman's parents to express his desire to marry their daughter, as is common in Thailand, or a dowry, the property that a woman's parents give to a man's family in exchange for having their son marry her, as is common in Indian cultures. The Thai Royal Institute defines *sin sort* as follows:

> *sin sort*: n. money that a bridegroom gives to the parents of the woman he is about to marry, to constitute the *kha nam nom* (ค่าน้ำนม) "breast milk fee" [or fee for] rice fed [to her in her childhood]; (legal) money that a bridegroom gives to the parents, adoptive parents, or guardian of a woman, depending on the case, in exchange for the woman's consent to marry; (archaic) a bribe.[1]

Kha nam nom, or "breast milk fee," used in the definition above means money given by the bridegroom to the woman's parents or guardian for having brought her up, as in "Her parents did not ask for money, but I'm determined to give them some money as *kha nam nom*."[2]

There is uncertainty about the origins of the term *sin sort,* but it has clearly been a part of Thai society for a long time, as it is found in the following sections of the *Three Seals Law,* which King Rama I (r. 1782–1809) compiled from old Ayutthayan laws in 1804:

> **Article 106:** If any man who has asked for the hand of the daughter of any respected person has already given *sin sort* and arranged a *khan mak yai* (ขันหมาก ใหญ่) ritual procession, but the two [husband- and wife-to-be] are not yet living

together, should the man commit an indecency upon or against his wife[-to-be], who thereupon kills him, the wife[-to-be] shall be deemed innocent and the *khan mak, sin sort* and associated goods shall belong to the woman's parents.

Article 109, section 1: If a man has gone to ask for the daughter of any respected person to be his wedded wife and has already given *sin sort* but has not yet married the woman in an auspicious ceremony nor gone to live and sleep with the woman, should this man die, the respected person shall divide the *sin sort* into two parts: one part shall be returned to the man [sic], and the other part shall belong to the woman. If the woman dies, the *sin sort* shall belong to the woman's parents entirely. If the woman has already lost her virginity (*sia tua* เสียตัว) to the man, and the man dies, the *sin sort* shall be the woman's entirely, because it is *sin hua bua nang* (สินหัวบัวนาง) for the woman.[3]

Both articles show that *sin sort* was seen as proof of the man's intentions to stay with the woman. *Sin sort* was also a type of property for which the law could specify rightful owners in various kinds of cases. Whether sexual relations (*phet-samphan*) had taken place between the betrothed man and woman constituted part of the legal considerations, reflecting the woman's lack of rights over herself. The law stated that if the woman had been sexually violated (*thuk luang lamert thang-phet*) by the husband-to-be before the formal marriage ceremony had taken place, the *sin sort* went to her parents, because the woman was considered their property and therefore they had to be compensated for damage done to this property. Another legal article stated that if the couple had had sex, the woman was considered to be the man's wife as a result of that act, and should the man then die, the woman would be the recipient of his inheritance, in this case the bride price or *sin sort*. A woman engaged to a man did not yet have full wife's rights to inheritance, especially if she had not stayed with the man for a period specified by law.

Krommaluang Ratchaburidirekrit, also known as the father of modern Thai law, speculated that in the premodern period there were generally two ways for a man to gain a wife, either by abduction or purchase, and because the giving of *sin sort* is such an old tradition in the country, the latter was probably more typical of the people of Siam. He noted, "Engagement gold is much like money used to buy goods, and *sin sort* is the price a man pays for a woman."[4]

Specifying the value of *sin sort* was like determining the woman's price, further perpetuating the idea of women as property—the property of her parents before the wedding, the husband's property afterwards. Thus, a family asking for a high *sin sort* for a daughter was equivalent to publicly announcing that the woman in question was very valuable in terms of beauty, characteristics, and/or lineage. The dearer a woman's price, the more she was admired by society. The idea that a woman's value could be measured in money still survives in modern Thailand, although the idea of buying or selling a woman has given way to explanations that consider the value of *sin sort* as a measure of the parents' status.

In the days of Field Marshal Plaek Phibulsongkhram, Thailand's prime minister from 1938 to 1944, and again from 1948 to 1957, the custom of asking for high *sin sort* was seen as a social problem and an obstacle to nation-building. This was because the state had a policy of supporting marriage and childbearing, based on a belief that a larger population would make the nation greater. Thus, the state appealed to parents not to ask for high *sin sort*. However, this call seems to have been ineffective because the custom of asking for high *sin sort* remains common even today.

In Thai law, the old meaning of *sin sort* as a compensation to the parents of a bride for their efforts and expenses in raising their daughter has changed into seeing it as a price for the woman's consent to marry.[5] Its value is still negotiated between the parties involved. In northeastern Thailand this process is called *khat kha dorng* (คาดค่าดอง), "setting the price of becoming related." In the northeast, *kha dorng* means *sin sort,* and marriage is referred to as *kan kin dorng* (การกินดอง), "eating and being related," as the bride and groom's families become "related" (*dorng* ดอง) through it.

Sexual Inequality as Cultural Heritage

Many interpret the expression *sin sort* as consisting of *sin* (สิน), "property," that the man has to give to a woman's parents for them to permit him to *sort*(*sai*) (สอด[ใส่]), or "penetrate," that is, to legitimately have sex with the woman. While it is not clear if this was the term's original logic, existence of the custom clearly shows that society's expectations for men and women are different. The man is expected to be a leader and head of the family, while the woman is supposed to be a good homemaker for her husband and a good mother to their children. The man's quest to prove his leadership qualities begins when he decides to have a family. He will need to send an intermediary to negotiate the marriage with his bride-to-be's parents and then arrange money for *sin sort* and a *khan mak* procession. Later, he will show leadership by building a house. Women, on the other hand, are inculcated with the idea of being good wives and followers, which is demonstrated by respecting and trusting their husbands and keeping house to perfection. This fulfills the husband's high hopes for her, as evidenced by his taking the effort to arrange all the money for *sin sort*.

Sin sort not only reflects gender roles but also the sexualities linked to them, since marriage really boils down to societal permission for a man and a woman to legitimately have sex with each other. Thus, *sin sort* can be seen as the price the man pays for sex—to gain ownership rights over a woman's body. Accordingly, one of a good wife's duties is to satisfy the husband's sexual needs whenever he desires.

These deeply embedded sexual values were also reflected in previous Thai law that was devoid of any understanding of rights and sexual equality, such as article 276 of Thailand's Criminal Code, effective from 1956 to 2007, which did not acknowledge rape within marriage. This caused suffering to many women who had to endure sexual violence by their husbands in order to maintain their status as wives, whether due to economic dependency or to avoid being labeled as one whose family had broken down, or as a *mae mai* (แม่ม่าย), that is, "widow" or "divorcee," all of whom are still viewed with prejudice by society. Being labeled *mae mai* also constitutes a source of embarrassment for the woman, given the grand wedding and the showing off of a grandiose *sin sort,* which presumably both failed to guarantee a worry-free life together as a couple. In 2006, article 276 of the Criminal Code was changed to recognize rape within marriage as a crime. The former phrasing "whoever rapes a woman who is not his wife" became "whoever rapes another person" is legally liable to prosecution, to protect wives from being forced to have sex by their husbands. This change was, in part, due to long-term advocacy by women's rights groups.

Thai law does not recognize the registration of a marriage between two men, two women, or a man and a transgender woman. Nevertheless, many same-sex couples are divided categorically according to gender roles—in the sense that one party plays a masculine role and the other party plays a feminine role—as a result of their adhering to mainstream marriage ideology within their own relationships. This appropriation of sexual ideology constitutes a challenge to society to accept these relationships, by showing how they, too, follow the values and traditions of society. The appropriation of mainstream ideas of marriage and *sin sort* within Thailand's culture of women who love women is shown in the following web board posting by a self-identified *tom* talking about marriage plans with her *dee* partner:

I think I'll graduate, work, save enough money for the *sin sort* they ask for, buy a car, buy a house, buy everything my partner (*faen*) wants. I've been able to provide my partner with everything. But what should I do? In my partner's family, nobody likes me. And my family doesn't like her, either. I truly love her and hope to marry her. One more thing: my partner's dad doesn't like *toms*. Will he be able to accept me? Guess I won't ever see that day. But whatever happens, I'll make my dream come true.[6]

Sin sort is considered to be a sensitive matter, as it relates to attitudes and values toward love, gender, sexuality, money, and social class or status. A Thai marriage website states that disagreement regarding *sin sort* between the families involved in any marriage is quite likely, as in the case of a wealthy young man whose relationship with a woman had been good until her mother asked for an eight-digit *sin sort*. At this point, his parents told him that if he wanted to marry he had to arrange to pay the *sin sort* by himself. In another case, a bride worried that her husband-to-be would arrange a *sin sort* "inappropriate for his status," and that guests would be embarrassed when they discovered this on the wedding day. However, she did not dare tell this to him directly, lest he think badly of her. *Sin sort* can thus be a source of frustration for couples.[7] Forty years ago, the pop song *Sip meun* showed how one man felt when he was asked to pay a high *sin sort:*

I went to propose, because I had the money,
I'd worked for a year; I wanted to have a partner to take care of.
But oh, my heart, what I had to endure, no hope,
The money was not enough.
The dad-in-law was mean, selling for tens of thousands; mom-in-law smiled;
    myself, I was heart-broken.
Ten times ten thousand, ten times ten thousand, ten times ten thousand.
Ever so smiling, overjoyed, she would devour it.
Dear Father, I'm done. Dear Mother, I'm poor. Ten times ten thousand, it's too
    much for me.
I don't want to struggle against those who would sell their child.[8]

The delicacy of this issue is particularly clear in cases in which couples consist of a Thai bride and a foreign bridegroom, especially if the man comes from a country with no *sin sort* customs. This is reflected in the following web board post by a Thai woman planning to marry a foreign man:

Yesterday I talked with my partner about the Thai wedding ceremony. I told him, "Before you can marry a Thai girl, you've got to read up on Thai marriage customs," because he'd read just this little and was ... stunned. Because it's just all having to pay, pay, pay ... So I said to him, "Will you change your mind? Are you sure that you want to be with me?" He said, "Yes, be it as it may." But he didn't understand why he needed to give money to others. He said, "If we are to marry, we'd better get married in America," because he'll undoubtedly go bankrupt, if he pays hundreds of thousands.[9]

Many women's parents do not ask for *sin sort*. Some women's families even help by lending or giving the money, or a part of it, to the bridegroom, and when the ceremony is over, the parents give it back to the couple to use as starter capital for their married life.

The significance of *sin sort* seems to depend on attitudes and communication. It is important that the families involved reach an agreement because, if there is no communication or if attitudes clash, a conflict could result and become an obstacle to marriage. Most married women on the website referred to above say that their parents did not ask for *sin sort*—as long as the bridegroom arranged a traditional wedding ceremony—because they saw that get married in this way would make their children happy. Some women say their parents did not demand it, but they themselves did. Yet others say they paid it by themselves to follow tradition, even when not demanded, and for some it was a true problem, capable of putting a woman in an awkward position involving her partner and her parents.

When *Sin Sort* Does Not Bring (Sexual) Happiness

Conflicts related to *sin sort* may not be as violent in Thailand as conflicts over dowries sometimes are in India. In 2003, the Indian Minister of the Interior and the National Crime Records Bureau reported that in that year alone there were over six thousand deaths of women and girls related to dowry issues through suicide or violence. It is not clear, however, if this number includes cases of parents killing their daughters in anticipation of their inability to arrange dowry.[10] In a capitalist society, in which primary importance is given to money, this particular ancient Thai tradition has the effect of putting pressure on all parties involved to negotiate and arrange the money. This was demonstrated in the case of a nurse who was driven to suicide as a result of worrying that she would be unable to provide the money for her son's *sin sort*.[11] There are plenty of other cases not severe enough to make it to the news, but which involve conflict between the bride and the groom, the bride's family and the groom, or the bride and her own parents.

The sexual health implication of *sin sort*, when calculated in monetary terms, is that a marriage often results from economic considerations and becomes a match made to favor the social status or prestige of the families involved, rather than something that emerges from the couple's love for each other. Combined with a patriarchal relationship framework, it can make the wife unable to express her sexual needs or to negotiate consensual, safe, and enjoyable sex with her husband, which, in turn, can lead to the risk of STDs. It can also make the wife powerless to practice birth control and can even lead the husband to rape his wife.

Sin sort might also legitimize sexual violence in cases where a man first sexually violates a woman and then uses marriage involving *sin sort* as a way to avoid legal consequences, especially if he is infatuated with her and wants to tie her to himself, and if she herself cannot think of a better solution to maintain face and the reputation of her family. While a high *sin sort* might help save face, it cannot help the reluctant wife to protect herself from STDs, HIV/AIDS, or unwanted pregnancies.

The expression *sin sort* demonstrates that it is not a private matter for two persons to have sex or children, but rather requires full societal legitimacy. It also involves a number of people, and it involves power issues, from the personal level all the way up to national policies on population control. This ancient tradition illustrates and also perpetuates sexual values and norms that continue to involve inequalities, be it the man's duty to find money for *sin sort* or the expectations that the woman will be a good wife and mother, maintain harmonious relations within the family, and fulfill her husband's sexual needs. Hence, neither the fact that a woman today might be more knowledgeable or financially independent than was typical in the past, nor any other circumstance affecting why a couple marries, can be taken as a guarantee that both parties will have a safe and enjoyable sex life, as long as society still holds onto patriarchal notions in sexual matters, or only accepts sex within a monogamous, heterosexual marriage.

6 *HEUN* (หื่น): TO BE SEX-OBSESSED

Sulaiporn Chonwilai

Whence *Heun*?

The word *heun* (หื่น) is encountered both in spoken Thai and in the print media in Thailand, which often use it when reporting cases of rape and sexual violence. It is generally considered impolite because it is used to condemn persons who show signs of intense sexual desire too strong for them to avoid revealing their emotions and actions. *Heun* is used almost exclusively of men, hardly ever of women, either as a verb or an adjective, as seen in the following newspaper headlines:

- *Heun* son of village elder brutally rapes young woman—police successfully hunt down culprit.[1]
- Two *heun* teachers get fifty-year prison sentences for raping pupils.[2]

Sometimes the expression *heun kam* (หื่นกาม)—where *kam,* from the Pali/Sanskrit *kama* (sexual desire) means "sex"—is used to emphasize the explicitly sexual nature of the desire at issue.

The *Dictionary of the Royal Institute,* 1999 edition, defines *heun* as a verb: "having a strong urge (usually used of sexual desire [*kamarom*]),"[3] a meaning that totally parts ways with the expression *heun-han* (หื่นหรรษ์) used in poetry in the sense of being full of confidence, willing, merry, and appreciative. In northern Thailand, the word *heun* is considered vulgar, because it means copulation by animals. *Heun* evokes images of the lustful gaze of wild animals or humans— always male—preying on their victims, perhaps using violence to force them to have sex. Many young people today, however, use it in a playful way to describe their own feelings. Used in this way, it is not a very strong word, albeit considered a bit dirty. Used to explain others' behavior, it conveys blame, as when used by newspapers to refer to those accused of rape. Hence, its register depends on the context of its use.

Two other words have meanings similar to *heun*. *Krasan* (กระสัน) is defined as "to be sexually agitated" (among many other meanings) by the *Dictionary of the Royal Institute*, 1999 edition.[4] The origins of this usage go back to the poetic work *Lilit Phra Lo*. A second word, *ngian* (เงี่ยน), "to be horny," is a coarse term and hence not often used. Politely it could be expressed as "to want sexually," "to be sexually aroused," or "to feel lust." *Ngian* tends to be used to describe a man's behavior, and is not used to describe women.

Can Only Men Be *Heun*?

Because *heun* is related to sexual expressions and is quite a strong word, its use by the mass media when reporting on rape or sexual violence is equivalent to condemning the perpetrator as low class, sex-obsessed, perverted, or mentally ill, all of which are inferred from his inability to control his sexual urges. Its use also reflects the mass media's unrestrained power to judge by their choice of terminology whether a given action is right or wrong, good or evil. This is a situation that the accused person has no means of challenging. Using the word *heun* also supports the misconception that all rapists suffer from mental disorders or are sex-obsessed, because of what are represented as symptoms of *heun*. In fact, rape may take place for various reasons, and rapists have diverse class backgrounds and personality types. Most rapists are not mentally disturbed. Finally, reporters are rarely present when rape takes place to observe the details and then describe them graphically with the word *heun*. They use the word anyway, never considering the consequences.

That *heun* is used mostly of men reflects the Thai socio-sexual norm that allows only men to express their sexual desires or to be the active partners in sex. Words that describe women's behavior of the type that communicate their willingness to have sex tend to give an impression of an invitation to have sex rather than to be explicit expressions of the desire itself. Examples include *len hu len ta* (เล่นหู เล่นตา), "to flirt" (lit. "to play with the ears and eyes"), *hai tha* (ให้ท่า), "to flirt," *oi* (ออย) and *ran* (ร่าน), "to be lustful."

The use of *heun* also reflects the fact that while it is considered normal for men to express their feelings with coarse words, women—particularly unmarried, middle-class women—are not supposed to use impolite or sexually loaded words.

Women who express their sexual desires or openly talk about sex tend to be seen as sexually experienced, sex workers, or both. A woman who is thus perceived may be misunderstood as challenging, even inviting men to have sex with her, when, in fact, she is simply talking about sexual matters.

For young people, especially when chatting on the Internet, *heun* is not quite as strong a word as it is when it appears in print media. In this context, it is not just used in connection with men. The web board of a male-only high school once featured a posting titled: "Women and men: Who *heun* more?"[5] Replies to this posting reflected that, in this context, *heun,* defined as sexual arousal, is not just a male phenomenon. Different genders may express it in different ways, but men exhibit it more openly, and in this web discussion it was noted that people of other genders and sexualities also *heun.* One person wrote, "Women *heun* a little, men *heun* normally, *tut* (ตุ๊ด) [effeminate gays or trans-women] *heun* more, and gays *heun* just colossally."[6]

Heun lies halfway between ordinary sexual desire and taboo. Society generally accepts that *heun*-ness or expressions of sexual desire as an ordinary thing for men and for those whose genders and sexualities have been influenced by masculine gendering; for example, *gays* and *toms* (see chapters 13 and 12, respectively). Thai society perceives these groups as sex-obsessed, and their choice to engage in sex with people of the same sex is mainly based on a strong and indiscriminate desire to have sex. In this context, it is noteworthy that the early Thai academic and sexological term for "homosexuality," *rak-ruam-phet,* has a literal meaning of "to love to have sex." When these perceptions are coupled with a patriarchal society, it is no wonder that these genders, which seem to have been influenced by male values and behaviors in their identity construction, are openly linked to *heun*-ness.

Kathoeys are seen as another gender that *heun,* even though they are males who wish to be, and mentally are, women who reject masculinity in their character and expressions, with some even going as far as undergoing sex reassignment surgery to rid themselves of male sexual organs. Given that *heun* is typically linked to masculinity, it is then odd that *kathoeys* are also linked to *heun.* Or, in the case of *kathoeys, heun* is perhaps more of a case of desiring a man with whom to have sex, than looking to perform sex on men, as reported in the following news item:

> *Kathoeys* now turn to *heun* and rape: four "sissies next door" trick twelve-year-old boy into town outing—*kathoeys* brutally gang rape boy—[who] passes out on the bed![71]

Although *kathoeys* are seen as another type of woman or as imitating feminine characteristics, they are nevertheless portrayed as *heun*-ing or lusting after men in TV soap operas, comedy shows, and motion pictures. Given that women are not supposed to *heun,* these perceptions appear to contradict each other. Besides the point of view that all genders can *heun,* or express their sexual desires, this apparent contradiction can perhaps be explained by three facts, namely that *kathoeys* have grown up in a patriarchal society, that they have been brought up as boys, and that they have a diversity of sexualities, which society does not necessarily perceive. It is, in fact, not strange that *kathoeys* dare to express their sexual desires openly. After all, they are no different from men—or other genders for that matter—in this respect. The important point, however, is that *kathoeys, gays,* and *toms* should not be subject to generalizations as being prone to being *heun* or sexually violating other people.

Women's *Heun-ness*

On a website popular with teenagers, one posting asked the following: "Which ones do you want to avoid more: Women who *heun kam,* or women who are *raet* (แรด)?"[8] Most female and male respondents stated they would rather avoid *raet* women (see chapter 2) because they thought such women were the type to mess around with men without limits, whereas *heun* was seen as more of a case of emotions that emerge naturally. One respondent wrote: "I'd rather avoid *raet* people. Sometimes, when we're *raet,* we've got to see if we are also beautiful, or what we look like . . . but I wonder why women can't *heun*—that's nature as it was created."[9]

In modern-day societies, medical information is readily transmitted across borders, spreading various perspectives on sex, love, and sexual pleasure. Many middle-class women previously inhibited in sexual matters have been influenced by this openness and now dare to show their sexual desires more openly than ever before, in the belief that women have a right to pleasure through sex with their loved ones, partners, or husbands. Hence, it is natural that many women now dare to say they *heun,* by which they mean that they openly express their sexual feelings. However, it is still said half-jokingly rather than with full seriousness. Actually, *raet,* which is defined in the posting noted above as a promiscuous woman who has sex with an unlimited number of partners, and *heun,* which means to express one's sexual desires, raise two different issues and should not be compared. Nevertheless, the posting does show that women who have sexual needs and who express them can be more easily accepted than can women who change their partners regularly.

In sum, usage of the negatively loaded term *heun* touches upon many important issues concerning sex, gender, and sexuality. One such issue is the power media have and which they use to control the use of language and perpetuate many misunderstandings in society about the personality, social standing, and the gender of rapists. Additionally, gender issues arise in relation to how this term, on the one hand, is used for blaming men, but on the other, is also used among men to communicate sexual desire openly. In contrast, women are still discouraged from showing their sexual desire, as seen by the scarcity of words referring to women's open expression of sexual needs. Finally, the use of the word *heun* can perpetuate sexual prejudices against people who have genders or sexualities other than man or woman (e.g., *toms, gays, kathoeys*), on the basis of a perspective that only allows heterosexual relationships within monogamous marriages, in a context of patriarchy, and remains blind to the diversity of genders and sexualities to be found across these groups.

7 *PO* (โป๊): TO BE OBSCENE DUE TO NUDITY

Sulaiporn Chonwilai

From Filler Films to "Brother, Want Some Porn?"

The Thai word *po* (โป๊) comes from the Teochew Chinese *pow* (โป๊ว). Contrary to popular belief in Thailand, the original Teochew term is not related to pornography or to the English term "porn." Rather, its incidental connection with sexual matters began in the cinemas of Bangkok's Chinatown district, Yaowarat, where short porn films supplemented ordinary films that ran less than the average length. Such "filler" films, technically called *nang thi ao ma chai serm* (หนังที่เอา มาฉายเสริม), were colloquially known among Teochew Chinese theatre owners by the Thai-Chinese hybrid expression *nang pow* (หนังโป๊ว). Later, the Chinese pronunciation was "Thai-ified" to *nang po* (หนังโป๊), as the expression acquired its current meaning of "porn films."[1] *Ya pow* (ยาโป๊ว) originally meant tonics that were taken to strengthen the body, but this expression is now mostly understood to mean drugs that stimulate sexual potency.[2]

Po has been in the *Dictionary of the Royal Institute* since 1950, when it was simply defined as "to remedy that which is defective." Later, this meaning was contested as not matching the word's generally understood meaning, and so the revised 1982 edition includes a definition still accurate today:

> *po*: v., to remedy that which is defective, as in *ya po*; to make things that are still incomplete complete, as in "Put some *po* paint on that hole; before that, put some *po* cement into the hole;" (colloquial) adj. to be naked (*pleuay*) or somewhat naked, as in *rup po* (รูปโป๊), "porn image," with the intention to show certain organs that should be covered, as in *taeng-tua po* (แต่งตัวโป๊), "to dress revealingly."[3]

It is not clear when the term was first used to refer to sexually arousing materials, but it has been used in connection with print matter including books, magazines, picture albums, and cartoons, as well as electronic media, such as websites, VCDs, DVDs, and video clips. It is also used widely in everyday life when referring to clothing or speech that involves sexual matters, as well as nakedness that is sexually arousing and may lead to having sex.

Using *po* in the sexual context implies a negative, judgmental connotation, suggesting inappropriateness. Thai values tend to see sexual matters as private, and sex is seen as appropriate for procreation or for love within a monogamous marriage. Showing certain body parts, talking about sexual matters in public, or expressing sexual desire or enjoyment are considered inappropriate. Materials showing images of naked or half-naked men or women have been branded as "sexually provocative materials" (*seu yua-yu thang-phet* สื่อยั่วยุทางเพศ) and are considered by the Thai authorities to be the cause of sexual crime, and as a result, they, too, are criminalized. Vendors have to sell these materials covertly, whispering, "Hey brother, want some *po* (porn)?"

Almost synonymous with *po* is *ek* (เอกซ์), from the English letter "x." This term is based on the U.S. motion picture classification scheme of the past, according to which films considered unsuitable for viewers under the age of seventeen due to their violent or openly sexual content were labeled "X-rated." In the U.S., these films are now classified as "NC-17." *Ek* is defined by the *Royal Institute Dictionary of New Words* as follows:

> ***ek***: v. *po*, as in "*Ek* VCDs are shown without restraint;" "This woman dresses *ek*" (abbreviated from the English "X-rated").[4]

The following English loanwords in Thai are similar but have more positive connotations:

> ***sexy*** (เซ็กซี่): v., beautiful in a way that sexually attracts the opposite sex, as in "This woman dressed the most *sexy* in the event." "The latest male model was super-*sexy*."[5]

> ***nude*** (นู้ด): adj., naked, naked art.[6]

> ***erotic*** (อีโรติค): adj., related to love, lust, or sexual feelings.[7]

Nude tends to be used when referring to nakedness (*khwam-pleuay*) in art or aesthetics. Likewise, *erotic* is used in literary and cinema circles, with an emphasis on art, and the beauty of language. Both are more positive terms than *po* and tend to be used by educated, artistic people. Works of art described by the terms *nude* and *erotic* imply sexual content for the elevation of the mind, unlike *po* materials, which are for sexual titillation. *Sexy* is a word of appreciation for appearance, attire, or expressions, such as *sexy* eyes, or a mouth, gaze, or smile that is sexually attractive to the opposite, or the same, sex.

Just How Much?: When and How Something is Labeled *Po*?

Whether one's attire is *sexy* or *po,* and whether certain materials are *erotic* or *po,* can be endlessly contested, since definitions and interpretations are based on societal norms and values that are further reflected in individual attitudes, perspectives, and tastes. In premodern Thailand topless women were considered an ordinary matter, since all rural women wore the *jongkraben,* a single large piece of cloth that when folded looks somewhat like trousers, with a cloth tied around the breasts. Many older women or women with families did not bother with the latter, and went topless in public.[8] But in our era, the women who wear spaghetti-strap or strapless tops, or tops that expose the navel, or who wear see-through shirts that expose the nipples are considered rather *po* by many, and are criticized or condemned accordingly. For example, a young woman who wore an evening dress open on the sides from the chest down to the thighs when acting as a presenter in a national film awards ceremony was criticized and became big news, even prompting her educational institution to consider disciplinary action. But having found that she had worn underwear, the institution concluded that, "Although the dress looked too *po,* the young woman did not go to the extent of not wearing the lower part of her underwear."[9]

The basic right a person has to choose his or her own attire is, in practice, limited by sexual values and beliefs, such as *rak nuan sa-nguan tua* (see chapter 2), and the belief that by wearing revealing clothing, a woman entices men and perhaps invites sexual violence. In the eras of King Rama V (r. 1868–1910), King Rama VI (r. 1910–25), and the mid-twentieth century prime minister Field Marshal Plaek Phibulsongkhram, the Thai state attempted to control its citizens' dress. For both men and women, going topless was seen as uncivilized, rather than seductive, and thus required intervention to bring it into line with Western standards of so-called "civilization."[10]

In whichever context, and however or by whomever, *po* is defined, women are the ones for whom *po* is most a matter of control, a control that extends over their bodies and sexualities. On many occasions, men can go topless without it being seen as strange or indecent, and it may even be seen as good-looking and sexy among Thais if they reveal muscular upper bodies or hairy chests. However, the same level of nudity (unless art-related) in women would be condemned inappropriate. Many women have to be constantly on the watch not to dress too *po* lest they be seen as a so-called "bad woman" (*phu-ying chua*).

Po materials (e.g., videos, magazines) are produced for heterosexual men, with the emphasis on penetrative sex between a man and a woman. They portray a woman's role as that of a mere sex object, whose purpose is to satisfy male sexual fantasies. Heterosexual relationships have a clear division of gender roles; namely, men must be the so-called active party and have sexual expertise, and the woman must let the man perform the act and satisfy his needs. Heterosexual sex is considered complete when penetration and ejaculation by the man have taken place. Viewers of *po* films may have little opportunity to know if the woman has experienced a climax or enjoyed the act.

Issues of *po*-ness, as nakedness, and *po* materials reflect the fact that society appreciates men more than women. As a result, men are given more opportunities to uncover their bodies and express their sexual needs than women are. Society controls women's bodies and sexualities through a framework of ideals that constitute what it means to be a good woman, including such aspects as covering up her body, not allowing herself to be easily touched, not expressing her sexual feelings, not looking for sexual experiences, and not consuming *po* materials.

Po-ness and *po* materials also reflect body-related beliefs regarding the ideal size or features of certain organs. Some of these cultural attitudes have been confirmed scientifically, e.g., the existence of certain places in our bodies, especially in the sex organs, which are easily stimulated and cause sexual arousal when touched. However, some beliefs do not have this kind of backing, yet, nonetheless, affect most people's sexual values and behavior. A good example is the belief that a big penis or large breasts will greatly enhance sexual pleasure for both parties.

The sexualities portrayed in *po* materials take sexual fantasies of non-mainstream, forbidden, or repressed behaviors and process them into images, such as those of rape, group sex, *swinging* (see chapter 20), pedophilia, zoophilia, or sado-masochism. Such materials are labeled *seu lamok anajan* (สื่อลามกอนาจาร),

"obscene publications," precisely because they portray images of these non-mainstream sexualities. They are considered inappropriate and are said to seduce, lead to sex obsessions, encourage sexual activity among youth who are still too young, and promote non-mainstream types of sex or sexual violence.

The sexualities of men who love men (*chai rak chai*) are also non-mainstream, but are nonetheless treated with increasing openness in Thai society today. They have also been influenced by the values that determine what is considered sexually attractive or arousing in a male body. Both heterosexual women and men who love men are infatuated with the masculine anatomy, be it a strong, muscular body, a big penis, or a round, tight bottom. While individual tastes vary, *po* materials produced for men who love men still emphasize big penises and sex acts with ejaculation as the climax, much like such materials produced for heterosexual men.

Although others might see *po* materials that portray sex between men as unnatural, contrary to tradition, or somehow baser than its heterosexual counterpart,[11] for men who love men they are a source of knowledge and experience, a supplement or an outlet for sexual fantasies that they are unable to fulfill in their everyday lives. Perhaps these materials, or the perspectives that men who love men have on naked male bodies, cannot be compared with those of women, because the socialization of women, which involves a devaluation of their sexual desire, means that even in the realm of the imagination, many cannot escape the narrow framework that society has set out for them. In contrast, social values that link maleness with open acknowledgement of sexual desire permits men who love men, like their heterosexual peers, access to a much less restricted, perhaps even unlimited, sexual imagination.

Obscenity vs. Imagining Sexual Pleasure

However much society attempts to ban or hide *po* materials, human sexual curiosity and supporting market mechanisms are likely to keep them available. Perspectives that view these materials as a reflection of Thai sexual values or as a variable in sexual health are less often encountered than the typical views that consider these materials immoral, as if they urge young people to have sex or lead to sexual crime. Two important questions arise:

- Are *po* materials merely obscene publications serving the abnormal sexual needs of certain groups?
- Does the presentation of *sexy* images of naked women really arouse men sexually to such an extent that they cannot control themselves?

If the answer to the first question is yes, most men's sexual needs can be considered abnormal, because almost every man (and many women) probably has had some experience with *po* magazines and VCDs, and for many these materials were their first sex educator (both theoretically and practically). Historian and columnist Nidhi Eoseewong, who admits that he, among many others, has benefited from *po* materials, discusses whether *po* materials lead to sexual violence, recognizing that what are called "sexual perversions" depend on psychological factors that are more complex than the materials themselves. He notes that "most people (including senior male members of the cabinet), upon seeing these materials, don't think of raping anyone."[12]

When considering *po*-ness from the perspective of sexual health, the question arises as to whether young women who dress in a *sexy* way (and thus clash with traditional Thai values) might simply feel proud of their bodies. It is hardly likely that anyone really dresses with an intention to provoke men to rape them. However, beliefs legitimized by pseudo-scientific explanations of men's supposedly uncontrollable sex drives entrap women under patriarchal power, meaning that they cannot dress as they like or go wherever they like, thus forcing them to feel afraid of being raped or of being seen as what are called "bad women." Husbands sometimes use violence against their wives out of jealousy when their wives dress in a *po* way.

Seen from a sexual health perspective, *po* materials facilitate sexual fantasies and liberate long-repressed emotions. They can also teach youth about sex in a life-like manner, if coupled with advice from adults. Many young men say they have learnt more about the purpose and use of condoms from *po* movies than from their classrooms, receiving answers to questions they dared not ask anyone. Adults—including both heterosexuals and homosexuals, men and women— also gain sexual experience from these materials, as well as a way to gain sexual pleasure through masturbation, pleasure that is safe with no risk of STDs, does not require buying sexual services, and so on.

In a society that treats sexual matters negatively and views them as matters to be covered up, people secretively consume *po* materials in great quantity. Sex without love and sex for pleasure (not procreation) are seen as inferior to sex within a monogamous marriage. Sex that is not penetrative and/or not what is considered normal (e.g., sex between persons of the same sex, oral or anal sex, masturbation, group sex, sex involving sado-masochism, etc.) is particularly condemned, even when mutually consensual. *Po* materials, whether homosexual or heterosexual, help open societal space for these non-mainstream sexualities, help create sexual fantasies, and also fulfill them in a way that does not expose the subject to societal alienation (e.g., masturbation in private).

However, most *po* materials still emphasize men's sexual pleasure. Viewers might think women portrayed in these materials enjoy the acts shown, but really the women shown in them are only representations, images of the kind of woman men would like to see, and are provided to allow men to reach their sexual goals. Very few *po* materials pay attention to women's feelings or aim to facilitate their sexual fantasies. These issues reflect a sexual inequality based on values and beliefs that men have a higher sex drive (thus requiring more outlets) than women do, that men are natural leaders in sexual matters, and that women should merely receive and meet men's sexual needs. It is thus not strange that men, whether homosexual or heterosexual, can survey the bounds of their imagination, learning about, and looking for sexual experiences more easily than can women. This inequality is the real source of many invisible sexual problems.

Po-ness and *po* materials are examples of challenges posed to the traditional sexual framework. These materials invite people to see taboo matters more liberally, and to learn about and try to imagine different types of sexual needs from their own. If these materials are seen as creative and educational instead of taboo, and permitted for all genders and sexual tastes, sexual pressure within society will be reduced, and more understanding between different genders and more acceptance of sexual diversity will result.

PART 2

SEXUAL PHYSIOLOGY

8 *HEE* (หี): CUNT

Monruedee Laphimon

A Word Most Thai People Dare Not Utter

The female sex organs have numerous names in Thai. These names reflect societal beliefs on sexual matters, especially women's sexuality, and are bound tightly to ideas about femininity. One term for the female sex organs is particularly taboo, and should not be uttered in public. It is *hee* (หี). Academic definitions of *hee* link it to the body and the anatomical process of reproduction. For example, the *Dictionary of the Royal Institute*, 1999 edition, defines it as: "*hee*, n. the reproductive organs of women or the females of some animals."[1] Sexual and reproductive health materials use the formal academic expression *awaiyawa seup-phan* (อวัยวะสืบพันธุ์), "reproductive organs," instead of *hee*, as in, "to have wound in the *awaiyawa seup-phan*."[2] Thai *Wikipedia* classifies *hee* as a biological term, stating that it is a Thai word for a sexual organ, and refers to further information under entries such as *awaiyawa seup-phan ying* (อวัยวะสืบพันธุ์หญิง), "female reproductive organs" and *chorng sangwat* (ช่องสังวาส), "vulva." According to Thai *Wikipedia*:

> *Hee* is a coarse (*yap*) word that refers to the female reproductive organs (*awaiyawa seup-phan ying*), which incorporate the *pak mot luk* (ปากมดลูก), "cervix," and *chorng khlort* (ช่องคลอด), "vagina" [lit. birth canal]. But the word is usually used in reference to the *chorng sangwat* (ช่องสังวาส), "vulva," or *chorng khlort*, "vagina," respectively, or to both of these together, but not including the *pak mot luk*, "cervix," or *mot luk* (มดลูก), "uterus."[3]

Anatomically, *hee* refers to the female sex organs, including the external organs, which consist of *khaem lek* (แคมเล็ก), "labia minora," at the mouth of the vagina, *khaem yai* (แคมใหญ่), "labia majora," larger than the labia minora and outside of them, and the clitoris, which is button-like and inside, as well as the internal organs, including *pak khorng thor patsawa* (ปากของท่อปัสสาวะ), "urethral opening," and *pak khorng chorng khlort* (ปากของช่องคลอด) "vaginal [birth canal] opening." The *chorng sangwat*, "vulva," and *chorng khlort*, "vagina," are interlinking structures, like the mouth and the throat. There is also a pink membrane covering the vagina, called *yeua phrommajan* (เยื่อพรหมจรรย์) or *yeua phrommajari* (เยื่อพรหมจารี), which both translate as "hymen."

Anatomical descriptions of the female sex organs, as well as the tearing of the hymen when a woman first has sex, are laced with sexual prejudice and contribute to sexual ideologies repressing women's sexual expression. Coupled with traditions that define what it means to be a "good woman" (*kunlasatri*), they perpetuate the belief that a woman's highest value lies in maintaining her virginity until marriage, while a man who takes a woman's virginity is not seen as doing anything wrong. This set of concepts reduces women's opportunities to learn about sexual matters, leading them to lack basic sexual knowledge and experience. In cases where women have had previous sexual experience, their relationships with other men will be darkened by the fear that their current partner will find out about any previous ones.

Some Thai websites indicate that the Thai word *hee* may be derived from terms in Pali and Sanskrit. In Sanskrit, the word means "evil, lowly, coarse, not good" or as a verb root that denotes "to decay." In modern Thai, this term would seem to preserve some of its original negative connotations. Its meaning is the opposite of *khuay* (ควย), "cock" (see chapter 9), which is perhaps derived from *khuyaha* (คุยหะ), meaning "a secret place," or, in other words, the male sex organ. In Pali, the definition of *hee* is somewhat neutral. It is synonymous with *hina* (หีนา), *hin* (หีน), *hin* (หิน), *iti* (อิติ), and *hiti* (หิติ), which each translate as "to be small" or "a narrow passage,"[4] in contrast to *maha* (มหา) or *maha* (มะหะ), which means "to be big/great/large." In the sense of "to be small," the Pali-derived *hee* is found in a range of terms, such as Hinayana (หีนยาน), "the lesser path," which is another term for Theravada Buddhism, as well as in *hee ta* (หีตา), "tear duct," and *hee tao* (หีเต่า), "turtle's tail hair."[5] However, in modern Thai the negative connotations of the word *hee* have made it a coarse term that should not be spoken in public.

Judging the female sex organs to be lowlier or baser than those of males leads to a sexual hierarchy in which men are seen as leaders and women as followers. This value system both directly and indirectly decreases awareness of and mutual respect for human dignity. Awareness and respect for human dignity, if unhindered by sexual hierarchies, would create positively oriented learning about sexual matters and, in turn, facilitate the equality of human beings and of sexual behavior free from prejudice.

Usually, *hee* is used in combination with other words to refer to unsatisfactory behavior (either sexually related or not) in both men and women. According to the Thai *Uncyclopedia*:

> **Hee** is a word of abuse referring to a man or a woman who lacks ability or is seen as lowly, using a comparison with lowly sex organs. Besides this, it is also used in expletives, such as *ai na hee* (ไอ้หน้าหี), "cuntface," *her hee* (เห่อหี), "cunt crazy," *hee haek* (หีแหก), "torn cunt," *phu-chai mi hee* (ผู้ชายมีหี), a "cunt of a man," and so on. It is also used together with other coarse words, such as in *jai thao hee mot* (ใจเท่า หีมด), "[to have] a heart the size of an ant's cunt," with a similar meaning to *port haek* (ปอดแหก), "to be cowardly," but much coarser and more broadly used, as in "This website's a real warrior site, and here's the supreme commander . . . don't come wasting my time, you ant cunt *(jai hee mot)*, skilled only with your mouth . . . show your phone number (if you dare)."[6]

Words of abuse that contain the word *hee* and which are used to refer to women generally denote female sexual behavior that is beyond the bounds of what is expected of a "good woman" *(phu-ying thi di)* or *kunlasatri* (กุลสตรี). For example, in northeastern Thailand the expression *hee khiao* (หีเคียว), "sickle cunt," suggests that the female sex organ is a sickle, reaping men as a sickle reaps rice. It is used for women who dare to express themselves sexually, have a strong temperament, wear revealing clothing, have many casual male friends, multiple boyfriends or husbands, or have sex with many men. In this it is comparable to *ran* (ร่าน), a "worthless, dishonorable woman." When *hee* is used in combination with *lae* (แหล่), "to be black" or "to be dark," as in *hee lae* (หีแหล่), it indicates a woman with black or darkly colored sex organs. This is said to identify a woman who is open about sexual matters, the presumption being that she has had so much sex her sexual organs have become dark, if not literally black.

In speaking with close friends, post-operative *kathoeys* or *sao praphet sorng* may refer to their surgically created neo-vaginas as *hee*, not considering this a coarse term or feeling embarrassed about using it. For example, a *kathoey* who would like to see the results of her transsexual friend's recent gender reassignment surgery might ask the friend quite openly, "Let me take a look at your *hee*" or "Come on, show me your *hee*."[7] In a *sao praphet sorng* discussion group one participant stated that "usually *kathoeys* use the word *hee* to verbally abuse women. We'll just add a few words to it to refer to women's bad, unseemly behavior."[8] Examples of *kathoeys'* terms of abuse for women include *ee hee wai* (อีหีไว) and *ee hee yort rian* (อีหียอดเหรียญ). In Central Thai *ee* (อี) is a pronoun that is used for women either by a person in a state of anger or when referring to a person of lower status, while *wai* means "to be fast/instant." Thus *ee hee wai* means "you fast/instant cunt" and is used to refer to women whose sexual behavior is considered bad, which is to say that they have many boyfriends. *Ee hee yort rian*, "you coin-op cunt," is quite a new expression, as Thai society has only recently become familiar with coin-operated machines. It refers to a woman who has sex in exchange for money.

Realms of Health and Media: Levels of Language

Thai newspapers tend to use the colloquial and curiosity arousing term *jim* (จิ๋ม) to refer to the female genitals when reporting on a crime, such as in the headline: "Weird sex—bottle stuffed into *jim* [woman] who dies."[9] The same news item also featured the term *chorng khlort*, "vagina," in the text and in a caption. This news item reported that an unidentified woman died of shock in a guesthouse on Soi Saphan Khu, Thung Mahamek Subdistrict, Sathorn District, Bangkok, after her male partner victimized her in a weird way by stuffing a beer bottle into her vagina (*chorng khlort*). This press item never used the term "sexual violation" (*kan-luang-lamert thang-phet*). Instead it described the deceased victim as "tomboyish" and the killer, a man, as her *khu kha* (คู่ขา), "casual sexual partner," who had a taste for intense sex (*rotsaniyom thang-phet run-raeng*).

With regard to publications focusing on health issues, such as those contained in the online library E-Lib, the expression *jut sorn-ren* (จุดซ่อนเร้น), "hidden spot," is used in addition to *chorng khlort* when giving advice about hygienic ways to clean the female sex organs, as well as the side-effects of using different vaginal cleaning solutions, the risks of STDs, and so on:

> Products for cleaning the *jut sorn-ren* should be selected with care, because the membranes in this part of the body are naturally thin, sensitive, and at risk of infection. What, in particular, should not be done is to spray water into the *chorng khlort*, because this might increase the risk of pelvic inflammatory diseases or, worse still, infection of the fallopian tubes, which might lead to ectopic pregnancy or sterility in the future.[10]

The Thai Health and Information Services website (www.thaihealth.net), which contains health information provided by medical doctors, uses the following terms for female sex organs:

awaiyawa seup-phan satri (อวัยวะสืบพันธุ์สตรี), "ladies' reproductive organs"

awaiyawa khorng phu-ying (อวัยวะของผู้หญิง), "women's organs"

awaiyawa phet phai-nork (อวัยวะเพศภายนอก), "external sexual organs"

awaiyawa phet (อวัยวะเพศ), "sexual organs"

chorng khlort, "the birth canal"

These terms often appear in information dealing with sexual organs and hygiene, in connection with topics like choosing underwear, the characteristics of the organs, and so on, as seen in the following excerpt from the Thai Health website:

Women's sexual organs (*awaiyawa phet*) are very creased and convoluted. Sweat, urine, or white discharge may get caught in the external organs (*awaiyawa phai-nork*), and if they are not kept clean correctly, yeast infection can occur and result in a bad smell or further infection. Thus, taking care of cleanliness is a good basic way to prevent abnormalities developing in the reproductive system. Women should thus take care to clean the external sexual organs (*awaiyawa phet phai-nork*) with soap and clean water each time when showering and then dry them from front to back, from the sexual organs to the anus, to prevent infection of the birth canal (*chorng khlort*) by bacteria from the anus.[11]

The various levels of language in this excerpt reflect the social class of the authors and the frame in which they view sexual matters. These variables are communicated implicitly by language, including the language used by other medical information publications, advertisements, the mass media, and so on. Although contemporary materials my increase women's interest in their own bodies and sexual organs by providing sexual hygiene information for women, including publications that use the expression *jut sorn-ren*, "the hidden spot," society, on the other hand, often describes the female sexual organs with terms associated with the fragrance of flowers. Women, too, often use these more euphemistic terms, for example, by comparing their vaginas to the smell of a rose. These terminologies are a hidden influence in women's lives, controlling the way they express the femininity of their bodies.

The socialization of women through the use of the *kunlasatri*, or "genteel lady," ideology makes women afraid of getting to know their sexual organs, at least until they face symptoms that force them to seek the advice of a medical professional who can examine these organs. The medical field thus confronts traditional morals and opens up a space for creating familiarity with female sex organs. Unfortunately, medical terminology itself is often presented through old clichés, such as the ability or inability to produce offspring and women's anatomical vulnerability to infections and sexual violence.

New Knowledge, New Meanings: Mechanisms of Resistance and Negotiation

In an article posted on a women's website, women's sexual organs are referred to as *awaiyawa suan ni* (อวัยวะส่วนนี้), "these organs," *awaiyawa phet ying* (อวัยวะเพศหญิง), "woman's sexual organs," and *norng jim* (น้องจิ๋ม), "younger sibling *jim*," as excerpted below:

> We can start surveying the female body straight away. Take a look at where the *clitoris* [English used here] is, what your labia (*khaem lek* and *khaem yai*) are like, and learn where different parts of the female sexual organs (*awaiyawa phet ying*) are located, such as the cervix (*pak mot luk*) . . . A perfect *norng jim* cannot be found in this world. Those ever so beautiful female sex organs (*awaiyawa phet ying*) exist only in porn magazines, and even there only as a result of airbrushing the photos. These organs (*awaiyawa suan ni*) in women differ from person to person. There is no prototype of "normal." What makes them different is the difference in the size and thickness of the labia (*khaem lek* and *khaem yai*), and the size of the *clitoris*. They're not the same in any given two persons. If you worry about this, try asking your lover (*khu-rak*) or a trusted friend. When you have heard the answer, you'll understand that all women are unique in this regard.[12]

This information shatters the illusion, often spread by pornography, that there is a standard appearance for all *jim*. In contrast, it suggests that women should feel pride in their sexual organs and get to know these organs by touching them. It also facilitates communication about women's sexual organs with partners and friends. Many readers have commented and shared their experiences, as in the following posting:

I'm lucky because my partner (*faen*) takes care of me as if I were a child. He cuts my pubic hair, bathes me, and massages me down there. I had to have surgery on my *jim*, and he was the person to clean the wound. He loves me so much. Whenever we have sex he also licks my *jim* every time. He's never despised it, but he makes love ever so hard (*raeng mak*) . . . Sometimes I like it, sometimes it hurts, but he usually asks how I like to do it and ensures that I feel excited and satisfied every time. I really feel it all the way up in me, all of it. But I like to rock on his thing, because it's big and long, and sexy, and rocking on it is so hot (*man*) and exciting.[13]

This posting not only reflects how the man took care of the hygiene and appearance of his female partner's sexual organs but also shows its author's resistance to the "proper woman" (*phu-ying riap-roi*) ideological frame in many respects, namely, her open communication on sexual matters with her partner, her readiness to disclose details of sexual acts, her expression of her own sexual tastes, and the pleasure she receives from sex. Nonetheless, her posting still perpetuates the cliché that a man's size matters in increasing a woman's sexual pleasure.

A debate was arranged on one website to decide whether *ju* (จู๋), a man's "willy," or *jim*, a woman's "fanny"(UK)/"pussy"(US), was the more powerful. The party arguing for *jim*'s superiority made these five arguments:

(1) *Quantitative superiority*: the *jim* is bigger and can enclose a man's *ju* entirely; (2) *Forcefulness*: the *jim* can constrict a *ju* until the latter is powerless; (3) *Efficiency*: a *jim* can reach a climax (*jut sut-yort*) [see chapter 16] a greater number of times than a *ju* can; (4) *Strategic superiority*: a *jim* can still give pleasure after having reached a climax through its contractions; and (5) *Anatomical superiority*: because a *ju* hangs outside the body, it is vulnerable to the use of force, but this is not the case with *jim*.[14]

These humorous arguments reflect attempts at creating new cultural meanings, based on the anatomical explanation that a woman's *jim* is not weak, but rather is powerful, efficient in achieving sexual pleasure, and not simply receptive but also capable of constricting a man's *ju*.

Diverse Terms: Sociocultural Meanings in Action

The diverse expressions and terms for the female sex organs include: *awaiyawa seup-phan ying, awaiyawa phet ying, chorng khlort, chorng sangwat, jim*, and *jut sorn-ren*. To this list can be added *khorng sa-nguan* (ของสงวน), "reserved goods," and even *yoni* (โยนี), "female genitals," which are typically used in educational materials, academic articles, and in the media. *Taet* (แตด), which really means the clitoris, and *pum krasan* (ปุ่มกระสัน) also tend to be used for female genitalia in general. *Thi lap* (ที่ลับ), "a secret place,"[15] is also used, as in "Young women have a new fashion: not wearing underwear and doing highlights on the pubic hair of their *thi lap*. This is a subject of widespread criticism at the moment."[16]

It could be said that academic texts on health care and language usage have also contributed to people choosing to avoid the use of the word *hee*, since it is regarded as a negatively loaded, impolite term. Instead, a wide range of euphemisms is used in addition to the terms already mentioned, such as words that reflect the anatomy of the organs, including *ru* (รู), "hole," *tham* (ถ้ำ), "cave," *rorng* (ร่อง), "furrow or groove," *klip* (กลีบ), "petal," and *khok* (โคก), "hillock;" euphemistic expressions that include metaphors for sexual anatomy and words denoting love or romance, such as *nern sawat* (เนินสวาท), "love hill," *rorng sawat* (ร่องสวาท), "love furrow," and *umong sawat* (อุโมงค์สวาท), "love tunnel;" expressions that refer to the organs' location in the woman's body, such as *chuang lang (khorng phu-ying)* (ช่วงล่าง [ของผู้หญิง]), "(women's) lower parts," and *trong nan (khorng phu-ying)* (ตรงนั้น [ของผู้หญิง]), "(women's) right down there;" and words comparing female organs with an animal, such as *hoi* (หอย), "shellfish."

Other euphemistic expressions contain words used in a religio-spiritual context, such as *yoni, thi lap*, or *khorng lap* (ของลับ), "secret thing," as in the following:

> *Yoni* means the base on which a phallic *shivalinga* is erected, considered a symbol of the female sex. Ancient Hindu textbooks state that both *yoni* and *shivalinga* are seen as the root cause of continual reproduction, but *yoni* is a force that facilitates power and greatness.[17]

The use of the expression *khorng lap* is also exemplified by the following comment posted to a web-board discussion:

> What the fortuneteller said [was] that I have moles or birthmarks on my *khorng lap* . . . Just what [parts of the body] does the fortuneteller mean by *khorng lap*?

Because any spot that one should not brag about or show to anyone in a public place can be a *thi lap* or *khorng lap*. Don't believe in fortunetelling too much. Watch out . . . if the fortuneteller wants to see your "hidden things" (*khorng lap*) in a "hidden place" (*thi lap*), it's a big issue . . .[18]

Words expressing the value and privacy of the sexual organs, and indicating that they should not be revealed include *suan nan* (ส่วนนั้น), "that part," *khorng sa-nguan* (*phu-ying*) (ของสงวน [ผู้หญิง]), "(women's) reserved goods," *khorng* (ของ), "thing," and *jut sorn-ren*, as in the following newspaper headlines:

- Witch doctor caught on the spot—made young woman strip in *long na* ceremony and groped her *khorng sa-nguan*.[19]
- Nine cruel sixth graders push female pupil to ground—use Scotch tape to close mouth—grope breasts and *khorng sa-nguan* feverishly right there in the classroom![20]
- "Ice" ever so sexy! Wow! Only asks to cover *khorng sa-nguan*.[21]
- True or false? Women who've had sex have a smell in their *jut sorn-ren*.[22]

Words that make comparisons between food smells and those of women's sexual organs include *kapi, pi, ee pi* (กะปิ, ปิ๊, อีปิ๊), each of which denotes "shrimp paste;" *khoey* (เคย), which denotes a paste made with baby shrimp; *pet* (เป็ด), meaning "duck;" and *pla khem* (ปลาเค็ม), "salted fish." Sorajak Siriborirak notes that:

What the Central Thai call *kapi* . . . the Nakhorn Sri Thammarat folks in Southern Thailand call *khoey*. But for Songkhla people, *khoey* means *khorng sa-nguan phu-ying* (women's reserved goods), which Nakhorn Sri Thammarat folks, in turn, colloquially call *pet*. Thus, having to refer to these things often causes confusion.[23]

Additional euphemisms include terms that reflect the organs' commercial value, realizable through sex work, as in the idiom *thi na pheun noi* (ที่นาผืนน้อย), "a small rice paddy," which compares the female sex organs to a place of work, and words that express the (small) size, delicacy, or adorableness of the female sex organs—implying that they should be taken good care of—or, alternatively, the youthfulness of the owner, such as *jim, norng jim*, the related *nu jim* (หนูจิ๋ม) and *ji* (จิ๋), or *norng sao* (น้องสาว), "little sister," as found in this web posting:

O, thin, clear condom, put it on the willy (*ju*). Don't be silly and put it into the *jim*. That will close the hole, the *hoi* will rot, and the little lady will really be left without... and when your *jim* itches, to be sure you've got to scratch it. If you are in the bedroom or bathroom that is private and out of other people's sight, and you spread your legs and scratch your *jim*, it won't bother anyone.[24]

In both colloquial Thai and the field of anatomy, the word *hee* is turned into a secret, hidden thing, and women can thus become estranged from their sexual organs. For example, in a workshop arranged by the Thai Women and HIV/AIDS Task Force in October 2005 in Nong Khai in northeastern Thailand, participants were advised to use a mirror to look at their *hee* in order to learn about their anatomy. Many participants said that one needs one mirror for the face and another one for the *hee*, as it was not appropriate to use a mirror that had been placed between a woman's legs to look at other parts of the body. Words such as *hee* reflect the coarseness or politeness of terminology that is directly related to how Thais are socialized into believing certain things. The euphemisms for *hee* carry hidden power and connote sexual repression, as well as women's attempts to resist these forces. They also tell us once more that language equals power, a power that labels male anatomy as superior to female anatomy.

9 *KHUAY* (ควย): COCK

Monruedee Laphimon

The Word, Its Origins, and Its Meaning: A Legitimate Sexuality

The *Dictionary of the Royal Institute*, 1999 edition, defines the word *khuay* (ควย) as "the reproductive organ of the human male or male animals of some species."[1] Thai *Wikipedia* defines it as the "male reproductive organs" (*awaiyawa seup-phan chai* อวัยวะสืบพันธุ์ชาย) and provides the following gloss:

> *khuay*: The reproductive organs of male living beings, functioning to procreate, to perpetuate the species. Consisting of both external and internal structures, but usually reference to them tends to be understood as including only the external structures. These external structures are: *ongkhachat* (องคชาต),[2] "the penis;" *antha* (อัณทะ), "the testicles;" *torm sang nam liang asuji* (ต่อมสร้างน้ำเลี้ยงอสุจิ), "seminal vesicles," which produce the semen that nourishes sperm cells; *torm luk mak* (ต่อมลูกหมาก), "the prostate gland," which functions to create a mildly alkaline substance to adjust the acidity of the vagina and to create a white substance to strengthen the sperm, increase their mobility, and enable them to pass through the urinary tract, blended with seminal fluid; and *torm Cowper* (ต่อมคาวเปอร์), "Cowper's gland," a tiny gland below the prostate, which functions to create a viscous secretion to lubricate the urinary tract.[3]

The Thai *Uncyclopedia* speculates that the term *khuay* was adapted from *khuyha* (คุยห) and *khuhya* (คุหย), which in Sanskrit mean "to be secret."[4] It may also be related to the term *phra khuyhathan* (พระคุยหฐาน), which means a man's "private parts" (*awaiyawa thi-lap*).

Khuay is typically used to refer to a part of the male sexual and reproductive organs (*awaiyawa phet seup-phan khorng chai* อวัยวะเพศสืบพันธุ์ของชาย) and is generally considered a vulgar, impolite word that is not to be used in public. Usually, the expressions *awaiyawa phet chai* (อวัยวะเพศชาย), "male sex organs," or *ongkhachat*, "penis," are used instead in formal, academic, or medical contexts, as in the following:

> The male reproductive system consists of two main organs: the testicles (*antha*) and male sex organ (*awaiyawa phet chai*). As the reproductive and urinary systems are close by and work together . . . a cross-sectional picture of the male sex organ, penis (*awaiyawa phet chai, ongkhachat*) shows that it is elongated in shape, located outside of the body on the front side, and functions as a conduit of urine and sexual fluids or semen (*nam kam* น้ำกาม) . . . Sexual arousal makes the penis (*ongkhachat*) stiffen, to permit its insertion into the vagina (*chorng khlort*) of a female. At the tip of the *ongkhachat* there is a neural hub, sensitive to sexual stimulation, comparable to the clitoris of the female. According to statistics, Thai men have *awaiyawa phet* with a mean erect length of five inches.[5]

The Royal Institute Dictionary of New Words lists a long group of words with meanings similar to *khuay* or *awaiyawa phet chai*:

ju (จู๋): "willy," also *ai ju* (ไอ้จู๋) and *kraju* (กระจู๋), both of which mean "willy"[6]

norng chai (น้องชาย): "younger brother"[7]

jiao (เจี๊ยว): "willy," also *krajiao, ai jiao*, e.g., *jiao* means *nok* (นก—lit. bird; met. a synonym for *jiao*); often used for a boy's sexual organ[8]

nok-khao (นกเขา): a "dove." The expression *nok khao mai khan* (นกเขาไม่ขัน), "the dove doesn't coo," denotes impotence, as in the following example, "Stress may cause *nok khao mai khan* in men."[9]

nok-krajork kin nam (นกกระจอกกินน้ำ): "a sparrow drinks water," and its synonym *nok-krajork mai than kin nam* (นกกระจอกไม่ทันกินน้ำ), "a sparrow isn't fast enough to drink water," denote premature ejaculation, as in the following: "They gossip that Somchai belongs to the *nok-krajork kin nam* group, and so his wife has a lover" [or] "She justifies having a secret lover on the basis that her husband suffers from *nok-krajork mai than kin nam* and is unable to make her fully happy."[10]

Newspapers use other terms, such as *jao lok* (เจ้าโลก), "lord of the world," and *hua maeo* (หัวแมว), "cat's head," and sometimes *phuang sawan* (พวงสวรรค์), "heavenly bunch," with this latter expression describing the bunch-like shape of the testicles (*antha*) or "balls" (*khai* ไข่ — "eggs"), but is nonetheless used to refer to both the penis and testicles together.

In Thai cultural beliefs the male's sex organ must have the ability to maintain an erection for a long time during intercourse, be able to engage in intercourse for a long time without ejaculating, and be big. The intercourse in question should be vaginal penetration by the penis for the purpose of procreation. Use of the word *khuay* and its synonyms often implies that boys' sexual organs are cute and adorable. While adult men's sexual organs are represented as being powerful in many ways, their condition depends on the age and health status of their owner. They need to be used and maintained carefully to avoid damage to their health and potency. Male supremacy over women is reproduced by paired expressions like *phi ju norng jim* (พี่จู๋ น้องจิ๋ม), "elder sibling Willy, younger sibling Fanny." Other terms imply that the male sex organs are secret and that sexual matters are mysterious and should not be disclosed.

Terminology of Thailand's Gay Culture: Penetrating the Societal Framework in Sexual Matters

A Thai *gay* terminology website lists words relating to the male sex organ and divides them into three groups: words referring to appearance, words referring to size, and words referring to the use of the male sex organ, as follows:

Words relating to the appearance of the male sex organ:

- **K.** (เค): n. The exact reason that Thai *gays* choose to use the English letter K as a slang term for penis is not known, but it is likely to be an abbreviation of the romanized spelling of *khuay*.[11]
- **mai** (ไม้): "wood," "stick."

Words expressing the size of the male sex organ:

- **hor mok** (ห่อหมก): n. a Thai dish of steamed fish with curry paste, wrapped into a small package of banana leaves. This idiom denotes a large penis that is clearly visible through a man's trousers. It is the opposite of *taep* (see below).

- **beum, tum** (บึ้ม, ตู้ม): adj. both of these are onomatopoetic words for the sound of an explosion and are used as adjectives meaning "big." They are used with *K.*, as in *K. beum!* "What a big cock!"
- **fu** (ฟู): adj. meaning to be enlarged into full size. It is used with *K.*, as in "*K. fu*" (เคฟู), an "erect penis."
- **alang, alangkan** (อลัง, อลังการ): adj. "attractive," "decorated," "large and pleasing to the eyes." It is used with K., as in *K. alang!* (เคอลัง), "gorgeous cock."

Words referring to the use of the male sex organ, and whether to hide it or not during oral sex:

- **klum taep** (กลุ่มแต๊บ): idiom. "a group that keeps the penis modestly, not letting it bulge." It is used when speaking of pre-operative transsexuals, who may seek to hide their penis (*taep*) when cross-dressing or trying to pass as women.[12]

The use of the English letter K. by Thai *gays* reflects their urban, middle-class characteristics. Some terms reflect the diversity of identities found among men who love men, as well as their sexual practices, creating new perspectives on sex that are not limited to the idea of sex for procreation only. The words that Thai men who love men have created to refer to the male sex organs also convey sexual matters in the context of sexual pleasure. However, the influence of traditional sexual values and meanings, namely, that sexual matters are limited to having sex, is still clearly visible. For example, in the emphasis that *gays* put on the size of the penis and in the comparison made between it and objects (e.g., *mai*, lit. a "stick"), which might obscure understanding of a male sexual partner as a real person rather than just the owner of a desirable penis.

Ham . . . Khlam . . . Khuay:
Usages Specific to Social Groups, Regions, and the Internet

Khlam (ขลำ), a synonym of *khuay*, is equally vulgar. Websites that compile slang terms, like Thai *Uncyclopedia*, state that *khlam* was originally a Northern Thai word with two meanings: "(1) used as a noun, it means the male sex organs (*awaiyawa phet chai*), typically used for small boys; and (2) used as an adjective, it means stupid, inauspicious, unlucky, very bad, wicked, not good, indecent, or injurious (when used of food)."[13] The term *khlam* has spread among teenagers on the Internet because a red, wormlike, almost penis-like monster was given the name *khlam daeng* (ขลำแดง), "red *khlam*," in the popular online game *Ragnarok*. Among teenagers the term also has two types of usage. As a noun, it means the male sex organ, as in *khlam hak* (ขลำหัก), to have a "broken-off penis," or to cut off a guy's *khlam* and turn him into a "eunuch." As an adjective, it means "very bad," as in "Today was . . . really *khlam*."[14] It is also widely used as an interjection that refers to silliness or inappropriateness. It is used like the close homonym *kham* (ขำ), "to be funny," in slang.

In northeastern Thailand, *khuay* refers not only to the male sex organ, but also means "water buffalo," which in Central Thai is pronounced *khwai*, as noted in the following Internet posting:

> I have to ask for everyone's forgiveness. I've no intention to speak coarsely, but I wish to expand on this topic. The word *khuay* in the Northeast means *khwai* (ควาย), "water buffalo." So, don't misunderstand. Let's see an example of the usage of the word *khuay* in Northeastern Thai . . . "When your *khuay* gives birth, don't forget to keep the afterbirth . . . I like soup made of water buffalo afterbirth."[15]

Used as a swear word, usually by men, the speaker might say *khuay* or *khuay oey* (ควยเอ๊ย), "Oh, *khuay*!" or just raise his middle finger without directing it at anyone or anything in particular, to vent his emotions in an unpleasant situation, or use the word when speaking with close friends. Using *bak khuay* (บักควย) or *ee khuay* (อีควย), as words of abuse in northeastern Thailand, is considered very coarse, comparable to Central Thai expletives like *ai ngo* (ไอ้โง่), "you fuckwit!," *ai wen* (ไอ้เวร), "damn you!," *ai sat* (ไอ้สัตว์), "you animal," *ai khuay* (ไอ้ควย) or *khuay oey*, "you dickhead," *samorng ma* (สมองหมา), "you dog brain," and *panya khuay* (ปัญญาควย), "you dickhead/fuckwit." In Central Thai, *ee*, denoting women or effeminate men, and *ai*, denoting men or masculine women, are used often as derogatory particles before invectives.

Ham in Northeastern Thai not only means a man's "eggs" (*khai*), i.e., "balls" or "testicles," but also denotes the penis as well. *Bak ham noi* (บักหำน้อย), "little balls," is an old Northeastern Thai expression that refers endearingly to a young boy, but it is now very rarely used. This is because while being endearing in some contexts, it can also be seen as derogatory, especially if the speaker is not someone familiar to or respected by the listener.

Since the word *khuay* is banned on most Thai websites as being obscene, people resort to various tricks to avoid it being spotted by the system, such as changing the final consonant symbol, adding various symbols into the word, intentionally misspelling it, or pressing the Shift key on some letters, which turns them into other letters when using the Thai keyboard.

Evolution of Language: Taking Issue with Power

Because *khuay* is impolite, other words tend to be used instead. Their meanings have to be interpreted mostly by context and the speaker's tone of voice, including words for official and medical use, such as "male sex organs" (*awaiyawa phet chai*), "male reproductive organs" (*awaiyawa seup-phan chai*), and "penis" (*ongkhachat*), as in the following excerpt from a medical text:

> Having sex is not forbidden, except in the case of cancer in . . . the male reproductive organ (*awaiyawa seup-phan chai*), in which case the doctor will give individual advice.[16]

In addition to official and medical terms, there are words that specify the size of the male sexual organ and are thereby linked to power inequalities, such as *jao lok*, "lord of the world," *mangkorn* (มังกร), "dragon," *chang noi* (ช้างน้อย), "little elephant," *hua maeo*, "cat's head," and *nok*, "bird," as well as words that relate to the adorableness and age of the owner of the male sex organ, such as *ju*, *norng ju*, *jao jampi* (เจ้าจำปี), "lord *jampi*," *jampi* being a kind of flower; *jiao*, *krajiao*, *ai jorn* (ไอ้จ้อน), and *krapok* (กระโปก), all meaning "scrotum," and *ai jiao plorm* (ไอ้เจี๊ยวปลอม), a "fake willy."[17] The following quotation from a website providing advice on circumcision shows examples of "cute" references to boys' sexual organs:

> The issue of children's genitals, a boy's *ju* "willy" and a girl's *jim* "fanny"/"pussy," is very important, especially when it comes to a small son's *klorng duang jai* (กล่องดวงใจ), "dear little tube," which is an issue that many parents wonder about in terms of whether or not they should have their son circumcised (*khlip*). . . . Circumcision has traditionally been practiced among Muslims according to Islamic principles, but recently a trend has emerged among some parents who are not Muslim to have their newborn sons circumcised, because they believe that

this will help improve the hygiene of the boy's *jao jampi*, make cleaning it easier, prevent bacterial infection, and reduce the risk of cancer.[18]

Other less impolite terms for *khuay* include words that portray the male organ as being loved, as something that should not be exposed, as private property and valuable, such as *khorng lap phu-chai* (ของลับผู้ชาย), "a man's secret thing," *ai nan (khorng phu-chai)* (ไอ้นั่น[ของผู้ชาย]), "that thing (of a man)," *tua diao an diao (khorng phu-chai)* (ตัวเดียวอันเดียว[ของผู้ชาย]), "(a man's) one and only," and *norng chai*, "little brother."

Then there are words that express the benefits the owner can expect from using his sexual organ for intercourse, such as *thaeng hareuhan* (แท่งหฤหรรษ์), "joystick," as well as words that are used in religious and spiritual contexts, communicating sacredness, such as *leung* (ลึงค์), "lingam," and *hua leung* (หัวลึงค์), "lingam head," and words that denote the shape of the penis, such as *thorn leung* (ท่อนลึงค์), "lingam tube," *thaeng leung* (แท่งลึงค์), "lingam stick," and *thaeng ai tim* (แท่งไอติม), "ice cream stick." Other words to describe the penis include those that are based on the characteristics of the testicles, such as *luk antha* (ลูกอัณฑะ), "testicles," *khai* (ไข่), "eggs," and *phuang sawan*, "the family jewels" (lit. "heavenly bunch").

Additional synonyms for *khuay* include metaphorical words connoting efficiency, aggression, and violence, such as *peun* (ปืน), "gun," and *dap* (ดาบ), "sword,"[19] as in the following posting to a web discussion on oral sex:

> Something that should be watched out for is firing your gun (*peun*) accidentally while in action, because whenever you shoot your gun by accident, the determination and stimulation that let you take your partner to the highest pleasure will be gone. Take her up onto the shore first and then you'll reach land yourself.[20]

Finally, regional terms, such as *ham, khlam, khai nui* (ไข่นุ้ย), *dor* (ดอ), and *krador* (กระดอ), and English loanwords, such as *dildo* (ดิลโด) are often used instead of the term *khuay*.[21]

Leung . . . Palat khik: The Language of Power

Siwaleung (ศิวลึงค์), "Shivalinga," is a phallus-shaped symbol used in Brahmanism and Hinduism that expresses abundance and the god Shiva's powers of creation. It is considered the spiritual source of the male sex (*ong kamnert phet chai*

องค์กำเนิดเพศชาย). Shivalinga worship came to Thailand with Brahmanism. Shivalinga-shaped talismans are also hung from the waist to protect against the goddess Kali. In Thai, they are called *palat khik* (ปลัดขิก) and mimic the shape of a circumcised penis that has had the foreskin removed.[22] Phitthaya Bunnag states that worship of *palat khik*, sometimes also referred to as *khunphet* (ขุนเพ็ด) or *ongkhachat*, has been practiced in Thailand since the Ayutthayan era.[23] They were used to give protection to young boys, especially those who were sickly or believed to be at risk of attack from malevolent spirits. Boys wore *palat khik* from a thread around their waist, which was thought to trick malevolent spirits into believing that a young boy was really a powerful, adult man who should be avoided. Traditionally, the *palat khik* was fastened to a boy's waist so that it hung down as close as possible to his own sex organ. Made of auspicious wood, coral, horn, or ivory, *palat khik* were consecrated by Buddhist monks in order to make them more powerful.

The origins of the word *khik* are still uncertain, but it is likely to have been a Central Thai word for penis that has since fallen out of use, due to it having been perceived as vulgar. It was then replaced with the Pali term *khuyha*, which, in turn, became the contemporary Thai term *khuay*, which, in its own turn, became a coarse, taboo word.

The function of *palat khik* has shifted from a spirit-tricking tool into a talisman to be worshipped to bring good luck. People tend to take a *palat khik* to a shrine when they pray for the well-being of a male child, or else they touch products they intend to sell with a *palat khik* in order to improve sales. This act is accompanied with incantations involving the word *hee*, "cunt," to trick malevolent spirits into believing the products are worthless and so not worth stealing. Here are two examples of such *palat khik* incantations or mantras of the Buddhist monk Phra Suan of Chachoengsao Province:

Ohm. Rich, mighty rich. Thirty-two cocks (*khuay*) encircle the cunt (*hee*). Sell quickly, sell well, tear the cunt (*hee*) apart, go home. *Ha ha ha* (This should be chanted in full in a single breath without stopping).

Ohm. O *khlik* (ขลิก—cf. *khik*), O *khlak* [ขลัก—cf. *khik*]. Snapped hook, crooked hook. O tail, which tail? Men like *hee*, women like *khuay*, makes me ever so rich (*ram ruay*). Smack head, smack head, smack head.

In chapter 8 it was noted that a humorous debate was arranged on a website to decide whether a "willy" (*ju*) or a "fanny"/"pussy" (*jim*) is more powerful, that is, the "real lord of the world" (*jao lok tua jing*).²⁴ Those arguing that a willy (*ju*) is more powerful stated:

(1) *Quantitatively:* A willy (*ju*) can pierce a fanny/pussy (*jim*) and cause injury, and a willy can also penetrate an arse (*tut* ตูด) . . . (2) *In terms of efficiency:* a fanny/pussy is wide like an ocean, does not constrict a willy, and a willy can also hide its troops inside a fanny/pussy to make trouble nine months later . . . (3) *In terms of power:* oftentimes a willy reaches a climax, while a fanny/pussy doesn't . . . (4) *Strategically:* exhaustion of a willy means victory has already been achieved, and still allows for more sex if the owner of the fanny/pussy doesn't call the owner of the willy an uncle . . . (5) *Anatomically:* not every willy hangs down—in some men it is so long they have to wrap it around the waist—and when in the cinema a fanny/pussy is not secure, a naughty hand might bother it . . . (6) *Magically:* a willy is the symbol of greatness, as in *leung* and *palat khik.*²⁵

The above debate, from the perspective of a willy (*ju*), and also the history of *palat khik*, repeats the notion that men are superior to women. The debate also reflects Thai thinking on certain sexual matters; for example, the idea that men can freely choose their sexuality (they can choose whether to penetrate either women or men), male sex organs are the center of the sexual universe, sex between men and women is aimed at making the woman pregnant (which reflects the man's potency), and that it is more important for a man to achieve orgasm than it is for a woman. Men are also represented as the source of women's anxiety about sexual violence. All this reflects the construction of beliefs and values that see the male organ as supreme, and the birth of a male child as an achievement. It also reflects Thai society's complicity in allowing sexual exploitation to take place, violating the principle that peaceful coexistence in society should be based on equal sexual relations.

10 *EUM* (อิ่ม): TO BE BUSTY

Monruedee Laphimon

Eum: A Term with Uncertain Origins

Eum (อิ่ม) is a contemporary word that refers to the female breasts. The *Royal Institute Dictionary of New Words*, which collates new words previously unlisted in the Institute's official dictionary, defines it as:

> **eum**: n. large breasts, as in, "Before she started work in the entertainment industry, she enlarged her *eum*." v. to have large breasts, as in "This superstar is really *eum* ... beautiful!"[1]

In the Matichon dictionary, *eum* is defined as a slang word and used as an adjective to mean a "busty, sexy, and attractive woman."[2] When *eum* was searched on Google (www.google.co.th), thirty-five pages of results containing over three hundred sites appeared. Random clicks on these links revealed a plethora of news items, articles, as well as beauty and health products, and spa and beauty clinic advertisements, such as "Just use this Perfect Lift cream, and you can say goodbye to flat *khai dao* (ไข่ดาว), 'fried egg,' breasts, which become *eum* straight away"[3] and "Change 'fried egg' *khai dao* breasts to *eum* in just four weeks."[4] Health and beauty articles also feature "secret food tips for increasing the *eum*-ness [of] breasts,"[5] and the like.

The Google search also revealed advice including a "method for increasing *eum* in order to wear a beautiful dress for a wedding,"[6] complete with illustrations and a step-by-step explanation of a method according to which the breasts are lifted by first attaching clear tape around the chest to make them seem fuller, and then applying foundation cream and eye shadow to accentuate the curves and the cleft between the breasts. However, the most common search result with the term *eum* was entertainment news about female superstars and their clothing, such as:

- Tata Young super-*eum*.[7]
- Yoga swan pose (*eum, ek*, super-*sexy*).[8]
- "But" [a male celebrity] dates girl, no less white, more *eum* than "Poey."[9]
- How to increase *eum* with lingerie.[10]

The web search also revealed many media sites that emphasize the marketing of women's sexiness, as in "white, beautiful, Chinese-looking, *eum*—from *Cute* magazine."[11] A dormitory of a famous university was nicknamed *ban a eum* (บ้านอะอึ๋ม), or "*Eum* house," in 1995, reflecting the residents' wish to welcome beautiful, cute, *eum* young women into the dormitory.[12]

There is no certainty as to who first used the term *eum* or when. In any case, it has been in wide circulation for some time in entertainment media and advertisements referring to the bodies or clothing of young female superstars and singers. Its use has also spread among the general public, teenagers, students, and businesses providing beauty enhancement services, such as cosmetic surgery, health, and nutrition products, as well as women's fashion clothing. Capitalism, print media, motion pictures, and music have disseminated meanings of *eum* to the public, without much questioning of the social mechanisms involved in creating the sexual values associated with the term—social mechanisms that control women's bodies by positioning them as there to please men. Reproducing beliefs, social norms, and a culture of *eum* in exchange for financial gain goes hand-in-hand with the consumption of values and beliefs related to women's value and bodies.

Eum-ness and So-called "Thai-style" Femininity

Valuing "big breasts" (*nom yai* นมใหญ่, *nom* meaning either "breast" or "milk" in Thai) is not a new phenomenon in Thai society. An ancient Chinese opus on physiognomy, which is the art of inferring a person's character from his or her appearance, was translated into Thai during the reign of King Rama I, and reads:

If the breasts are large, straight, and wide at their base, have red areolas and dark nipples, that person will have wealth, luck, and intelligence.

If the breasts are small, crooked, and pointed downwards, and have white areolas, that person cannot trust anyone, will have suffering, and die young.

If the areolas are wide, that person is brave, calm, and composed.

If the breasts and areolas are narrow, that person is foolish and has but little thought.[13]

Classical Thai literature and poetry also describe the beauty of breasts that are large and round, or large and close to each other, which is considered to reflect the influence of Indian values of feminine beauty, as illustrated in murals and statues at many historical sites.[14]

However, the concept *eum* also reflects the male gaze that evaluates women's bodies and pushes many women (as well as trans-women [*sao praphet sorng*] who desire feminine breasts) that are not naturally "busty" (*eum*) into attempting to increase their *eum*-ness (*khwam-eum*) with a plethora of oral or topical breast enlargement products, or through surgery. And yet, in an era when society values sexiness in both men and women, and women dare to reveal their bodies in public more than in the past, women with beautiful breasts (both natural and enlarged) like to exhibit them with pride, without seeing their bodies as sex objects for men.

Media of various types influence the values that emphasize women's beauty, be it images of swimming suit fashions or other fashions that are marketed by highlighting sexiness, erotica, nudity in men's magazines, films, soap operas, beauty contests, pictures of female superstars at various social functions, or fashion columns by columnists who are well-known for evaluating nude photographs, and so on. For example, a men's website evaluated the swimsuit models of a well-known women's magazine, using terminology with the same meaning as the word *eum*:

She is considered a woman whose whole body is full (*uap-at* อวบอัด) and firm. You could say that her body is balanced, yet she has enough to brag about to anyone, be it her tall and slender figure, her breasts that are full (*uap-im* อวบอิ่ม) and just the right size, or her ever so bulging buttocks that are simply begging to be fondled and that attract the gaze of many a young man.... It can be seen that the top-down perspective of the camera, focusing on that pair of mounds, guides our gaze down to her two breasty hills (*nern than an uap-im* เนินถันอันอวบอิ่ม) to our eyes' content. What could be more *uap-at*, round and grope-inviting than this?... There is no such thing in this world![15]

Uap-at means "to have abundant flesh, while also being firm and beautiful" and it is used in reference to young women, while *uap-im* has a similar meaning, "to have abundant flesh, to be beautiful."[16] Men tend to use the imagery-inducing terms *uap-at* and *uap-im* when describing and defining women's bodies and breasts, which they see as territory for the male sexual imagination and activities.

The word *eum* also reflects how sexual discourses operate on women's bodies through a belief and meaning system, which creates societal values about breasts (*tao nom/suang ok* เต้านม/ทรวงอก) as a source of feminine charm that stimulates men's sexual feelings/desires. *Eum* is very commonly used by the entertainment media when writing about women's bodies or the revealing clothing of female superstars, singers, models, or high-society women. News items with images showing the bustiness or *eum*-ness of young female superstars or news that reports their breast enlargement operations always sell well. For example, media have picked up on the enlarged breast size of several famous mixed ethnicity (*luk-khreung*) Thai-Caucasian singers by juxtaposing "before" and "after" pictures, and readers have wondered whether the breasts in the "after" picture are real or fake. When their owner responded that her large breasts were due to push-up techniques, numerous critics sprung up, stating that the woman in question had lost credibility:

It's good that she dares to express herself . . . but it's too sexy, and coupled with her exposed breasts during the show until you could almost see the nipples, and showing her bum too. . . . Well, it's like she's sold all of her body already. Now, it might be a leaked photo, but knowing there would be photographers, she still wore that . . . She should watch out a bit more; there are lots of paparazzi these days. She should behave in the cute way she did before. Or is she trying to up her ratings by showing her sexiness? Mmm, Thai women these days don't quite *rak nuan sa-nguan tua* [love and reserve their bodies] (but then again, she's only half Thai).[17]

The news about this "super-*eum*" singer reflects various perspectives on *eum*-ness within Thai society, such as individual rights, the role of medical technology in managing women's bodies, women's bodies and seduction, the structure of the capitalist economy, market mechanisms, the commercialization of women's bodies, media and its reflection of beliefs on gender and sexuality, and also the involvement of ideas of *rak nuan sa-nguan tua*, or chastity (see chapter 2), which is an ideal that young Thai women are supposed to strictly observe. Furthermore, the fact that the singer was not a hundred percent Thai was mentioned as if to reduce the harshness of the criticism of the superstar for revealing her body (contrary to what the ideology of *rak nuan sa-nguan tua* decrees for "real" Thai women), which reflects the fact that Thai society can compromise attitudes related to *eum*-ness when it comes to women who are perceived as "other" (*pen-eun*).

The so-called "super-*eum* singer" (*nak-rorng sao sut-eum*) phenomenon shows what beauty and sexiness are, at least according to the values and definitions transmitted and perpetuated by mainstream media. They are not limited to facial features but are also dependent on the size of the breasts (*na ok* หน้าอก/*tao nom*). Thus, women who are born with breasts (*na ok na jai* หน้าอกหน้าใจ) not as large as they or their social group would like are able, if they choose, to use technology to increase their sexiness and beauty.

While the main point of increasing one's *eum*-ness is to match contemporary definitions of beauty and sexiness, the *eum*-ness so created is nonetheless still seen as being inferior to its natural counterpart, quite like trans-women (*sao praphet sorng* สาวประเภทสอง), who have had sex reassignment surgery and are criticized as not being "real women" (*phu-ying jing*) since their sex organs can't be compared with those of so-called "genuine women" (*phu-ying thae thae*).

Eum-ness, Gender, and Well-being

In addition to the media, beauty enhancement businesses, including those offering cosmetic surgery, also play an important role in the creation of beliefs related to women's *eum*-ness, and also to that of transgender *sao praphet sorng*. For example, consider a beauty column in the Thai edition of *Cosmopolitan* that advised women to "show off their full (*uap-im*) cleavage." The column referred to an old scientific belief, now discredited, that large breasts are a result of the upper portion of the body imitating the roundness of the genital region.[18] It went on to recommend ways of scrubbing breast skin to make the breasts look fair-colored, using cosmetics to trick the eye to make the breasts seem large and firm, and using padded lingerie to make them seem round, firm, and erect. Today, leading women's magazines, entertainment magazines, and even family magazines that are popular among women are full of advertisements for clinics that provide cosmetic surgery, including breast enlargement and other cosmetic breast operations.

Thus, *eum*-ness, women's sexualities, and consumerism are inseparably linked. Women are expected to make themselves look good and sexy in the eyes of the opposite sex in order to meet patriarchal sexual tastes and values. Many women spend a lot of money on changing their bodies to feel satisfied about themselves, but, in fact, behind this satisfaction of the woman lies the husband or partner's satisfaction. Furthermore, if the clinic that a woman uses for these operations is substandard, she may face health hazards, but it seems that women generally focus more on the anticipated result than the possible risks.

Eum for Whom? . . . Why Does One Have to be *Eum*?

Many women strive for *eum*-ness to increase their self-confidence, to please their husbands or lovers, to obtain the feminine beauty certain professional occupations demand (e.g., stage and screen actresses, dancers, singers, TV presenters, etc.), or for other reasons. However, there is one group of women who attempt to do the opposite, namely, to have a flat chest. These women define themselves as *tom* (see chapter 12) and are seen as adopting a masculine role through clothing and expressions. Some websites for women who love women advertise products like breast binding cloths, specifically made for *toms*. *Toms* who bind their breasts usually state that they don't feel confident dressing in a masculine way if they have big breasts, especially if their breasts are as large or larger than those of their female partner. This matches well with the advertisements that tout benefits like "increasing confidence" or "reaching the firmness that *toms* want." Many *toms* insist on binding their breasts even if it leads to some difficulty with breathing, and even if they know that binding the breasts leads to a higher risk of breast cancer. They respond with various kinds of justifications, such as the following one from a women who love women website:

> Binding the breasts is a matter of personal preference. If someone asks why I do it, I've got to reply that it is for my own satisfaction and good feeling about not having large, bulging breasts. It's our own body shape and we may prefer to have it any given way, right? Some people have small breasts and want big ones, so they go for surgery. Some have big breasts and want small ones, so they go for surgery or bind them. It's not wrong in any way.[19]

Interestingly, many *toms* refuse to have large breasts or a busty *eum* look, but may well like women, or *dees,* who look *eum*, or would like their partner to look *eum* due to having been influenced by masculine or Western values.

In the past, Western society valued *eum* (or even overweight) women as the archetype of feminine beauty because these characteristics showed the woman had enough to eat, a high societal status, and was healthy. Consequently, *eum* was considered a sign of abundance. Later, values concerning women's beauty shifted in the West due to the influence of medicine, fashion, and the mass media. Now, to be seen as beautiful, women must not be overweight, both from an aesthetic point of view and because obesity is known to lead to various illnesses and many other problems. Although society now prefers slender women, it still values busty (*eum*) breasts as a sign of a woman's sexual attractiveness to men.

Values defining beauty and sexiness in Western fashion and entertainment circles have influenced those in similar Thai circles. Female superstars, both Thai and those of mixed Thai-Caucasian backgrounds (*luk-khreung*), now display their sexiness by wearing tight clothing or by exhibiting particular body parts as much as possible to increase their popularity. This can be seen from the frequent occurrence of leaked pictures of superstars at social events or fashion shows. Such news items usually attract many readers.

Once a survey was arranged to chart superstars' opinions as to whether showing one's *eum*-ness was a way for new faces to establish themselves in the entertainment circuit. Both male and female stars tended to reply similarly, namely, that dressing up to show one's *eum*-ness was an ordinary thing in contemporary society, but that the choice of dress should be appropriate for the occasion. Some said dressing to reveal *eum*-ness depended on the season (e.g., female stars having swimsuit photos taken in the summer), others said that it was a way to attract media interest, and yet others considered it a necessity dictated by the type of dress chosen by the team organizing a media event, not by the star herself. Some stars felt that dressing up in a sexy way was an individual right based on the person's taste and that those who chose sexy attire had probably already considered its appropriateness for themselves. Two male stars said that since they were men, they didn't feel it was much of an issue at all. They viewed it as customary, but also stated that Thai society didn't quite accept such attire and needed time to adapt to it.[20]

The above examples reflect a clash of contrasting Thai perspectives: on the one hand, the expectation that good women should not reveal their bodies too much in public, and on the other, the views of contemporary women who consider choice of dress to be one's right and a matter of personal taste, fashion, values, or modernity (*khwam-than-samai*).

Women's roles in the public sphere have gained importance and women today are more able than ever to work in a variety of occupations, just as men are. Many believe that women now have more freedom to control their bodies, as well as more sexual freedom. But under a sexual value system that emphasizes heterosexual, monogamous relationships and prioritizes male sexualities and operates within the context of global, borderless communications and a capitalist ideology, women's bodies are still under a male gaze. That gaze defines women's value, while at the same time the system commercializes women, primarily to meet men's needs. *Eum*-ness reflects these influences, and is an end goal that affects those born with female anatomy as well as those who want to change their bodies to acquire femininity. The pursuit of *eum*-ness illustrates not only that women's bodies are seen as sexual objects for men, but also that for many women pursuing *eum*-ness or increasing "bustiness" represents women's power to make decisions regarding their bodies, which can be considered as an investment to gain fame, fortune, or a lover.

From whichever perspective one considers it, society and women themselves should pay more attention to the possible adverse health consequences of medical procedures that are available for increasing *eum*-ness. Information available today tends to promote the commercial interests of the beauty industry businesses rather than provide women with information that is beneficial for their health. It is crucial that Thai society increase its base of knowledge on gender and sexuality topics to increase women's confidence, their appreciation of their sexual rights, and their understanding of the patriarchal ideas that operate through women's own attitudes, lifestyles, and behavior.

PART 3

SEXUAL IDENTITIES AND ROLES

MALE-TO-FEMALE TRANSGENDERS OR TRANSSEXUALS

Sulaiporn Chonwilai

A Longstanding Gender Identity

Kathoey (กะเทย) is the only term that refers to a gender identity other than man (*phu-chai*) or woman (*phu-ying*) that Thai society has long been familiar with and still uses. The term may have been borrowed from Khmer, or may be an original Thai word. This longstanding term has been used at least since the era of King Rama I, when the *Three Seals Law* (revised in 1804 CE) mentioned *kathoey* as one of thirty groups that were considered inappropriate for serving as witnesses in legal cases. This was because, according to beliefs current at the time, to be born a *kathoey* was seen as a karmic consequence of having committed adultery in a previous life.[1]

The term is also mentioned by the nineteenth-century Catholic bishop Jean-Baptiste Pallegoix, who in his 1896 *Dictionarium Linguae Thai* translated the term *kathoey* (then spelled กเทย) using the French and English word "hermaphrodite," which is a person with both male and female sexual organs.[2] The *Dictionary of the Siamese Language* published in 1855 by the American missionary the Reverend J. Caswell defined *kathoey* as "a person who is a man and a woman, and is called *khon kathoey* [*kathoey* person]." Published in 1873, the *Akharaphithansap* ("Word List") by the American Dr. Dan Bradley stated that a *kathoey* "is not a man, not a woman, [and] only has a urinary tract."[3] Similar words are also found in the Thai Ahom language, which uses *thoey*, and in Khmer, which uses *katoey*.[4]

The history of the word *kathoey* shows that Thai people have known of this phenomenon for a long time, and have viewed *kathoey* as people whose sexual organs differ from those of normative males and females, or who have hybrid male-female type sexual organs in the same way as those who are called "hermaphrodites" or "intersex" persons in English. Thai medical and psychological professionals later called such people *kathoey thae* (กะเทยแท้), "genuine *kathoey*."

Our research team collected information on older understandings of the meaning of *kathoey* by interviewing ten Thai senior citizens (five women aged sixty-three to eighty-one, and five men aged sixty-nine to seventy-four) at a cultural show at the National Museum of Thailand in Bangkok between November 30 and December 3, 2000. When discussing vocabulary related to people whose gender identity and sexuality differ from that of men and women, both the male and female senior citizens associated the word *kathoey* with "a man who wants to be a woman." A few of the older women also defined *kathoey* as "a woman who wants to be a man." Two of the interviewees mentioned "a person with both male and female sex organs" as a possible meaning. One said:

> In the past, *kathoey* meant that such a person had both male and female sexes (*phet thang chai ying*) in them. But now, it's not like that. Women want to be men; men want to be women. I don't know what to call them. If I were to call them *kathoey*, it would not be to the point, because a *kathoey* must have both male and female organs to match the word's meaning. I've seen and known one person like this before, when I lived in Nakhon Pathom, west of Bangkok. That person was in my group of friends and was my cousin, my uncle's child. At first, I didn't know that person was like that, but back then, aged fourteen, fifteen, in the countryside, when we were playing in the water, we were all naked, so I could see it [i.e., intersex characteristics]. That person has already passed away.[5]

Today, the *Dictionary of the Royal Institute Dictionary*, 1999 edition, still defines *kathoey* as "a person with both male and female sexual organs."[6] However, it also mentions, as alternative definitions, "a person whose mind and manners are opposite to their sex (*phet*)," and "a seedless fruit." Usually, people now have the second rather than the first of these definitions in mind when using the word *kathoey*. That is, they see *kathoey* as people born with male anatomy but whose appearance, manners, and sexual/gender identity are opposite to that which is expected of them as men.

Some forty to fifty years ago, before the present-day definition of the term *kathoey* became widespread, and before the terms *gay* and *tom* were introduced to Thai society, the term covered a variety of meanings. *Kathoey* was used to refer to a person:

- with both male and female sexual organs, or with indefinite sexual organs (i.e., intersex),
- whose behavior did not match their sexual organs, or rather a person whose behavior did not match the behavior society expected of a person with those types of sexual organs, (i.e., transgendered),
- who liked cross-dressing (i.e., a transvestite or cross-dresser), or
- who did not express himself or herself in cross-gender ways, but preferred a partner of the same sex (i.e., a homosexual person).

It is not surprising then that many Thai people still cannot distinguish between the meanings of the words *gay* and *kathoey*, because the word *kathoey* was previously used in reference to both identities that are gender-based (i.e., who one feels one is in terms of gender) and those that are sexuality-based, and reflect which gender(s) one prefers one's sexual partners to be. Besides this, the overlapping use of the words *gay* and *kathoey* in the past might also reflect class divisions among males with same-sex preferences. *Gay* was a new word, borrowed from English in the early 1960s and used to refer to males who had same-sex preferences, but who did not have a feminine mindset or any desire for feminine gender expression. The emergence of *gay* individuals was seen as a result of Western values and sexual culture being imported into Thai society. Being *gay* was seen as being mostly exclusive to Western-educated people and people who mingled with foreigners from the West, while the word *kathoey* was used to refer to people from all social classes, from the less-educated to the highest echelons of Thai society.

Over the past forty years, Thai society has gained familiarity with English-derived words reflecting same-sex identities and preferences, particularly the words *gay* and *tom*, which are increasingly used instead of *kathoey* to refer to male and female homosexuals, respectively. The word *gay* was introduced as a loanword and has a similar meaning as in Western societies, namely, that of a male who has a sexual preference for other males. The word *tom* was abbreviated from "*tom*boy," but its Thai definition differs from the Western one. In English, "tomboy" refers to a boyish girl, but in Thai the word *tom* refers to a woman who desires women more feminine than herself as sexual and romantic partners, who dresses as a man and/ or has a masculine gender expression. The increasing public presence of *kathoeys*, with both positive and negative media coverage, the linkage between *kathoeys* and expertise in certain lines of work (e.g., cabaret artists, beauticians, performing artists, singers), their public struggles for transgender and transsexual rights, and the fact that more and more *kathoeys* have presented their life histories in the public sphere, continue to shape the more specific, contemporary meaning of the term *kathoey*, denoting a male with a feminine mind, feminine characteristics, and a desire to be a woman. However, labeling a person of any gender/sex (*phet*) a *kathoey* is likely to make that person feel embarrassed or publicly ridiculed, because various medical, psychological, legal, cultural, religious, and media discourses legitimize only heterosexual, monogamous sex.

Today, Thai society tends to view *kathoeys* as being more feminine or more beautiful than those born with female physiology, to the extent that it fails to perceive that *kathoeys* are, in fact, diverse in terms of their gender identities and personalities, just like men and women are. *Kathoeys* are also used as selling points by entertainment media, and are often presented as overacting, sexually explicit, verbally caustic, and constantly man-hunting. Male actors are employed to play *kathoey* or female roles in films and TV soap operas. These phenomena contribute to the general portrayal of those whose gender or sexuality differs from the societal mainstream, as perverted (*wiparit phit-phet*), strange, amazing (*plaek pralat phitsadan*), or amusing (*na-khan*), and contributes to the discrimination they face throughout their lives.

From *Kathoey* to *Sao Praphet Sorng*: Kathoeys Defining Themselves

A posting on a *kathoey* or *sao praphet sorng* (สาวประเภทสอง), "second type of woman," web board (www.thailadyboyz.net) once asked what *kathoeys* themselves preferred to be called by other people.[7] Of the eighteen participants in the ensuing discussion, including the person who posted the initial entry, ten people expressed their feelings about being publicly labeled with the word *kathoey*. Seven stated that they could accept being labeled with this term, but three wrote that they did not feel very positive about it. One member of this latter group wrote, "Let's rather make it *sao praphet sorng*; it sounds pleasing to the ear. The word *kathoey* sounds so weird but, anyway, it depends on the way you say it."[8]

In Thai society people other than *kathoey* are so familiar with this term that they often overlook the sexual prejudice with which it is laced. The same situation pertains to the old term *pu mia* (ปู่เมีย), "man-woman," which is still used in the countryside. *Pu mia* is Northern Thai with a meaning similar to *kathoey*; *pu* means "male," while *mia* means "woman" or "wife." *Kathoey* themselves also use it as a self-referent term within their own community. However, several new terms have also emerged for males who express themselves in a feminine manner or desire to be a woman. These new terms include: *tut* (ตุ๊ด), *taeo* (แต๋ว), *Pratheuang* (ประเทือง), *krathiam* (กระเทียม lit. "garlic"), *norng toey* (น้องเตย "younger sibling Toey"), and *sao praphet sorng*. These terms can be divided into three main categories:

- Words with negative connotations used by outsiders to disparage transgender people and transsexuals, such as *tut*, *taeo*, or *Pratheuang*.
- Words that *kathoeys* use as self-referents, or are happy to let others use for them, such as *sao praphet sorng*, *TG* (from "TransGender"), or *ladyboy*.
- In-group words used by *kathoeys* amongst themselves to specify different shades of gender identity or social roles, such as *hua pok* (หัวโปก lit. "shaven head," for a *kathoey* who wears her hair short) or *kathoey khwai* (กะเทยควาย lit. "water buffalo *kathoey*" for a large-bodied *kathoey*), or different modalities of *kathoey* sexuality, such as *sao siap* (สาวเสียบ lit. "inserting girl," for *kathoey* who sexually penetrate male partners).

The word *tut* is an example of a term that *kathoey* typically do not like, or outright hate, because it is usually used derogatorily. Its origins may be traced to the 1980s Hollywood motion picture "Tootsie," whose lead male character of that name, performed by Dustin Hoffman, performed in drag. Some suggest that the word *tut* was already used before "Tootsie" was released, and claim that it comes from the English word "toots," an old slang word to refer to a woman, while others think that it may be a softened version of the Thai *tut* (ตูด), "ass" or "backside."[9]

In 1994, a punk-metal band named Sepia gained popularity by releasing a song titled *Kliat Tut* (I hate faggots) on an album with the same title. It expressed hatred toward *kathoeys* and used violent language, further perpetuating the negative ideas that Thai society holds about kathoeys and contributing toward legitimizing unashamed violence against *kathoeys* and homosexuals. Similarly, in 1998, pop singer Tai Thanawut released a song called *Pratheuang*, which ridiculed a *kathoey* called *Pratheuang*. This became the most famous pop song of that year. Non-*kathoey* people found the song very amusing, with the term *Pratheuang* itself quickly becoming a synonym for *kathoey*. However, *kathoeys* themselves do not like this disrespectful term.

Norng toey is an example of a term with no negative connotations. Like the word *krathiam*, it was probably created by slightly modifying the word *kathoey* to create an apparently more polite term—a common strategy in Thai language usage. The term *norng toey* communicates an endearing sense by drawing on the connotations of intimacy and cuteness associated with the word *norng* (น้อง) meaning a "younger sibling."[10]

Most *kathoeys* prefer to be called *sao praphet sorng* by outsiders, since this expression has a polite sense and does not have derogatory or disparaging connotations. It also matches the femininity and the desire to be a woman that *kathoeys* have. One contributor to a web-board discussion noted:

> As for the term *sao praphet sorng*—I feel it's a polite term for us. I wouldn't want ordinary people with ordinary genders (*phet pokati*) to call us *ai/ee tut* (ไอ้/อี ตุ๊ด —"damned faggot"), *krathoey* [alternative spelling of *kathoey*], *Pratheuang*, or the like. Perhaps because these words are short, blunt, and heart-piercing, most of us don't like them.[11]

When or by whom the term was first used is unclear, but the closely related term, *nang sao Siam praphet sorng* (นางสาวสยามประเภทสอง), "second category Miss Siam," was used in a 1972 news article on a *kathoey* beauty contest that was scheduled to be held in Lumpini Park in Bangkok. The Miss Siam Kathoey contest had to be cancelled after the police entered the event and ordered the contest and a *kathoey* fashion catwalk to be stopped, stating they were immoral.[12]

However, not all *kathoeys* like the phrase *sao praphet sorng*. Some question the necessity of a specific term. Those working on human rights issues, in particular, believe that the term creates a feeling of inequality or of being singled out as a category of second-class people. They think that it privileges those who see themselves as women, rather than as distinctly transgendered, and who desire a sex change and as such overlooks the specificity of *kathoey*-ness and its diversity. Many *kathoeys* do not desire a sex change and do not view themselves as women. Rather, they define themselves as *TG* or *transgender*, using the English acronym and term, instead of *sao praphet sorng*. *Kathoeys* may also refer to themselves as *ladyboys* when talking with English-speaking foreigners. This word may have first been introduced in the *kathoey* cabaret circuit. Many foreign sexuality researchers have also used the word *kathoey* (sometimes spelled *katoey*) as a label for one of Thai society's gender identities.

One more recent term that has been used to define *kathoey* is *phu-ying khamphet* (ผู้หญิงข้ามเพศ), literally "cross-gender woman" or "transgender woman." In 2007, this expression was used in political lobbying by the Transgender Women of Thailand group, led by a famous *kathoey* beauty contest winner, to permit *kathoeys* to use the personal title *nang sao* (นางสาว), "Miss," rather than "Mister"

(นาย nai), on their personal identity documents. It brought the rights of *kathoey* into the public eye once more, and the term itself was not particularly questioned because it was clear that it referred to a group of *kathoeys*.

Hua pok, *kathoey khwai*, and *sao siap* are examples of widely used words within *kathoey* and *gay* circles. They may have been further popularized by media and motion pictures with *kathoey* content. They reflect specific *kathoey* gender identities or sexualities. *Hua pok* refers to a young *kathoey* who cannot wear women's clothing or have long hair due to school regulations but who nevertheless has a so-called "sissy" (*ork sao*) gender expression. *Kathoey khwai* refers to a *kathoey* who has a big, muscular body, while *sao siap* refers to a *kathoey* who has a feminine appearance but who has not had sex reassignment surgery and who plays the insertive role in sex with a male partner.

Sao siap is a particularly meaning-laden word, as it shows that *kathoey* gender identity and sexual behavior or preference do not necessarily have to correspond. The usual perception is that a *kathoey*, or *sao praphet sorng*, is a woman in a male body who wishes to maximize her femininity, whether in terms of anatomy, manners, gender expression, or the sexual role she plays, and is the receptive party (*fai rap*) in penetrative sex, whether anal or vaginal (in post-operative cases). A *sao siap* has a feminine appearance and mannerisms, but she still has a male sexual organ and uses it to penetrate her partner, usually a male who identifies as a man (*phu-chai*), but sometimes a *gay* or another *kathoey*.

One person who plays the *sao siap* role explained in an interview given to the *Rainbow-Colored Way* radio program that she used to be just an ordinary *kathoey* who never thought of sexually penetrating anyone but subsequently felt like changing her image and sexual role.[13] She liked going to *gay* saunas, where *sao praphet sorng* are not well received by masculine-identified *gays*. When in a *gay* sauna, she had to downplay her femininity and she found many kinds of people approached her there for sex. Today she can play both the receptive (*fai rap*) and insertive (*fai ruk*) role, a sexual versatility that in Thai *gay* slang is called *both*, a word adopted from English. However, out of bed, she prefers a feminine role. On the radio program, she noted:

> When I was the sexually active (*ruk*) party for the first time, it felt like, oh, this is not "food" I've eaten before. I wasn't born for this. But when he turned his back to get a second round, I just pounded on. And the third round was pretty good. Nowadays, whichever type of guy approaches me, I can take it all—I don't give a damn. I've got a front and a back, so I'd best put them both to good use. . . .

Some people in the sauna have really curvy eyebrows—pretending masculinity to the max—but when we enter the private room, they turn their backs to me, and I've got to take them—hard! Sometimes I'm amazed at their guts. It's like, I'm finished [*set* "achieved orgasm"]—but just how much longer is it going to take before he moans that he has also come? Why do you have to pretend to me? You curvy eyebrows guy—you wanna be a man, you pretend you wanna take me, but take a look at your eyebrows—I'd better bang you instead.[14]

Today, use of the word *kathoey* conveys less prejudice than in the past, partly because the term is now more accepted as a self-definition word among *kathoeys*. But this does not mean that the general public understands *kathoeys* any better than in the past. It also does not mean that *kathoeys* are accepted as a gender equal to women or men, or that outsiders understand the differences between *gays* and *kathoeys* any better than before. This is clear from the discrimination that *kathoeys* and individuals who love the same sex (*bukkhon rak phet-diao-kan*) repeatedly have to face. For example, in 1997 the council of the Rajabhat Institute decreed that "sexually deviant individuals" (*bukkhon biang-ben thang-phet* บุคคลเบี่ยงเบน ทางเพศ) could not enroll in the institute as students, stating that such people were unsuitable as teachers. In 2000, the Government Public Relations Department asked producers to avoid presenting "third sex" (*phet thi-sam* เพศที่สาม) individuals in television programs, while in 2003, the permanent undersecretary for the Ministry of Culture stated that "sexually deviant individuals" (*bukkhon biang-ben thang-phet*) should not be allowed to become civil servants. In 2005, the Sexual Diversity Network challenged the Thai military's policy of labeling *kathoeys* in military draft sessions as persons afflicted with *rok jit* (โรคจิต), technically "psychosis" but often understood more broadly as "a psychological disease/ condition," and demanded a change in the terminology used. Most recently, we have seen activism by *sao praphet sorng* who feel that their rights are violated when they are not permitted to use a personal title on their identification cards and other official documents that matches their external feminine appearance.

Many more terms and expressions might emerge in the future to communicate *kathoey* sexual and gender identities. Even the meaning of the well-known old word *kathoey* has undergone historical shifts. The history of the term and of other related words not only reflects societal beliefs about sexual and gender identities in Thai society, which has long acknowledged the existence of people with identities other than man or woman, but also points to the power struggle each group engages in to define itself.

Yet outsiders still know *kathoeys* only superficially—by their external characteristics and their desire to express an identity contrary to their born sex—and fail to grasp the diversity in *kathoey* sexual lifestyles and other aspects of their identities. Most people still cannot distinguish between effeminate *gays* and transgender *kathoeys*. In this context, the desire of both *gays* and *kathoeys* not to be perceived as belonging to each other's group sometimes causes hostility between the two groups. *Kathoeys* who contradict societal expectations—such as those who are less feminine, have less than perfect looks or complexion, or who prefer the insertive role in sex—are rejected both by society at large and even by some of their *kathoey* peers.

Even more important than understanding the meaning and history of relevant terms is creating understanding and respect within society, both among *kathoeys* and outsiders, towards fluid and diverse sexualities. This is because prejudice toward those who have different sexualities or gender identities negatively affects the provision of health services that some *kathoeys* need in order to accomplish the physical changes they desire, whether through medicine, hormones, or other medical technologies. The health services sector should thus arrange for psychological support for *kathoeys* to promote increased self-acceptance and reduce stress and mental health problems. It should also provide accurate information to facilitate decision making with regard to sex reassignment procedures and information on the side effects of hormonal treatments, as well as providing specific services related to sexually transmitted diseases, the transmission of which depends on specific sexual practices within the group. Such services can only be created when society truly understands and accepts diverse gender identities and sexual behaviors.

12 *YING RAK YING* (หญิงรักหญิง): WOMEN WHO LOVE WOMEN

Sulaiporn Chonwilai

A Sexual Identity Defined by Women

Ying rak ying (หญิงรักหญิง) is a neologism created by combining easily understood, already existing Thai words, to refer to one type of women's sexuality. Its meaning is straightforward: a woman who likes or loves women and who may or may not have sexual relations with them. The term *ying rak ying* was born together with Anjaree, a group of women that has undertaken advocacy work to help society understand, accept, give importance to, and respect the rights of women who love other women. *Ying rak ying* has been the main term used in Anjaree's work for the rights of such women right from the beginning of the organization's activism.

Anjaree was established in 1986 and made itself known to the public in 1993. The name of the group was created by combining two Sanskrit/Pali words: *anya* (อัญญ), which means "to be other or to differ," and *jari* (จารี), which means "to travel or move." Together, these two words came to mean "to follow a different path" or "to travel a different way." Anjaree was established by four women's rights activists, all of whom liked women and had similar views on the rights of *ying rak ying*. They felt that Thai society still viewed *ying rak ying* as abnormal or sexually deviant, and that even groups working on women's issues did not pay attention to their identities or to women's right to love or have sexual relations with other women. Anjaree officially came out to the public in 1993 by sending a letter introducing the organization to "Uncle Go" of *Plaek* (Strange) magazine, which was the first Thai magazine to have a column on *gays*, *toms*, and *dees*.[14] Its first years were mainly spent increasing societal understanding on the rights of women who love women. Having successfully defeated the Rajabhat Institute's ban on what it called "sexually deviant students" in 2000 (see chapter 11), Anjaree expanded its scope to work for the rights of both male and female homosexuals, such as lobbying the Thai Ministry of Public Health to have homosexuality removed from the list of mental illnesses. The American Psychiatric Association announced the removal of homosexuality from the classification of mental illnesses and abnormalities in the United States in 1973, and in 1976 the American Psychological Association made a similar announcement, while the World Health Organization (WHO) removed homosexuality from the International Classification of Diseases in 1992. However, it was only in 2002 that the Thai Department of Mental Health, in response to Anjaree and a network of organizations campaigning on homosexuality, followed the WHO's decision on this issue and officially declassified homosexuality as a mental illness in Thailand.

One founding member of Anjaree said that the phrase *ying rak ying* was born of attempts to find a neutral self-definition term in Thai that was not enmeshed in sexual prejudice, in order to avoid the mistaken idea that being a woman-loving woman results from imitating Western culture or the adoption of Western values or beliefs. Besides the borrowed word *lesbian* (เลสเบี้ยน), which has negative connotations in the Thai context (see below), previously the only terms used to refer to the sexual identities of women who love women were the rather specific *tom* (ทอม), from the first syllable of the English "*tom*boy," and *dee* (ดี้), from the second syllable of the English word "la*dy*," which do not cover all groups of *ying rak ying*. The term *ying rak ying* was thus created to describe an identity with a straightforward, neutral, and unprejudiced meaning that would include all groups of women who love women and not emphasize sexual or gendered behavior alone. Anjaree has used the expression *ying rak ying* both among women who love women and also more widely and in its campaigns aimed at the general public. The term seems to have been received relatively well, as mass media now use it extensively.

Imitated Behavior or Concealed Identity?

While the term *ying rak ying* and the Anjaree organization are quite recent, sexual relations between women are not a new phenomenon in Thailand. Much historical evidence regarding them exists in the form of the term *len pheuan* (เล่น เพื่อน), "to play [with] a friend," which occurs in the Palatine Law (*Kot Monthian Ban*) text of King U Thong (r. 1351–69 CE) and which stipulated a penalty for royal concubines who were lovers. The term also occurs in an early Rattanakosin era octameter poem composed during the reign of King Rama III (r. 1824–51) on the relationship between two concubines. The expression was also used in King Mongkut's (r. 1851–68) commandment when he admonished his daughters, "Do not *len pheuan* with anyone; only have your husband." The expression *len pheuan* is a verb, referring to love or sexual relations between two women, and does not refer to the personalities, gender expression, or sexual identities of the women involved in any way.

While *len pheuan* was forbidden for the women of the royal court, and while there was a specific penalty for breaking the law, there is no evidence of a court lady ever having been punished for it. Perhaps Thai society has not considered sex between two women a serious enough issue to necessitate any concrete punishments. In the past, *kathoey* (กะเทย) was the only identity category for genders and sexualities, such as a man who wants to be a woman, a woman who wants to be a man, a person with incomplete sex organs, or a woman or man who does not want to change themselves to become the opposite sex but nonetheless loves and has sex with a person of their own sex (see chapter 11). All this shows that there has been sexual activity between persons of the same sex, whether men with men or women with women, but that it has not been paid attention to or accepted by society at large. Especially in the case of women, it has been seen as playing or acting according to a fashion, rather than as something genuine, and as something that could be changed by having more relations with men.

After World War II, Thai medical and psychological circles imported Western knowledge into their fields of study, which led to same-sex love being seen as an abnormality or sexual deviance and those with a homosexual identity or behavior as being perverted or *phit-phet* (ผิดเพศ), "wrong-sexed" or "wrong-gendered," as well as being violent, dangerous to society, and responsible for providing bad role models for young people. This attitude has forced women who love women to accept non-acceptance from society and makes them afraid to reveal their true identities to their families and others. Nowadays, Thai women who love women have more opportunities for being open about themselves than they did in the past. Due to activism by several NGOs advocating the human rights of homosexual people, these women are now more able to access information. However, the level of acceptance that *ying rak ying* receive in Thai society has not changed that much, and many women who love women might be out of the closet only within the *ying rak ying* community or among their friends, but still not have the courage to come out to their families.

From *Lesbian-Tom-Dee* to *Ying Rak Ying*: Diverse Identities?

Although the term *ying rak ying* has been used during the past ten years by the mass media and those advocating the rights of homosexual people, it is still not widespread or well-known within society at large. Nonetheless, there are many other words that are used to refer to women who love women but which have not been used in political activism, and which are better known within Thai society at large. Examples include *lesbian*, *tom*, and *dee*. All are derived from English, but their definitions in Thai are different from their English sources.

Lesbian (เลสเบี้ยน) means a woman who loves other women. While in English it is a neutral, non-derogatory term for women who love women, in Thai it is a word that *ying rak ying* do not use as a self-defining term. This is because it came into use in Thailand in the context of a system of psychological knowledge that labeled homosexuals as sexually abnormal or deviant. Psychiatrists, psychologists, the mass media, and academics in the field of sexology (*phet-seuksa*) are more likely to use the term *lesbian* than are *ying rak ying* themselves. For Thai people, the word also conjures up images of sex between women in pornography aimed at heterosexual men. Being an English word, it also lends itself to the misconception that the behaviors and identities of homosexual women are only found among middle class, urban women, as a result of adopting Western sexual values.

While the word *lesbian* has been used to define homosexual women by others, a section of this group prefers to define themselves as *tom*. This is a contraction of the word "*tom*boy," which in English means a girl with boyish behavior. However, in Thai, *tom* means a woman whose characteristics, expressions, and attire are close to those of a man, who loves the same sex, and who is the active/insertive partner (*fai ruk*) in sex. The word *tom* is thought to have been used as a self-defining term in Thailand from around the late 1960s or early 1970s. The beginnings of the study of sexual matters in Thailand dates back to the late 1950s, and the word *lesbian* was increasingly used in that era to explain what, back then, was called the sexual perversion (*kamawiparit*) of homosexuality in women. It has been suggested that masculine women who love women chose to use the word *tom* as a self-definition in order to avoid or to repudiate the negative and prejudicial meanings implied by the term *lesbian*. On the other hand, the word *tom* also seemed more modern than *kathoey*, the old word that represented a rough type of woman, matching the contemporary image *toms* present to society today. While the word *tom* was originally used among young, educated, urban, middle-class women, today it is widespread and well-known among both *ying* *rak ying* themselves and within society at large. The construction of *tom*-ness is linked to many ideas related to gender and sexuality. For example, it is thought that *toms* tend to pair up with *dees*.

Like *tom*, *dee* is a term of self-definition used to describe the gender and sexuality of a subset of women who love women, and it, too, is derived from an English word: "la*dy*." Unlike the English term, which refers to a polite or genteel woman, *dee* in Thai means a woman who has a *tom* as a partner, and who herself is no different from other women (*phu-ying*), other than in her sexual preference for *toms* rather than men. Typically, *dees* are sexually passive/receptive (*fai rap*). The word *dee* refers to sexuality rather than gender presentation, because a *dee* is only identifiable as a *dee* when she is seen with a *tom*, discloses she is a partner of a *tom*, or states that she likes *toms*.

Although *tom*-ness is more visible than *dee*-ness, and while *dee*-ness is only possible in the presence of *tom*-ness, Thai people in general conceive of woman-woman relationships as *tom-dee* relationships. This reflects the influence of a gender ideology based on binary opposites—masculinity vs. femininity—with *tom* as the representative of masculinity and *dee* as the representative of femininity.

Besides these terms, there are also other words referring to female same-sex behaviors or identities. Terms used by outsiders to refer to *ying rak ying*, or sexual activities between women, tend to be biased or derogatory, such as *ti ching* (ตี ฉิ่ง), "to beat cymbals," an expression that makes fun of sex between women. In northern Thailand the local term *pu* (ปู้), "male," is used to refer to women with masculine behaviors or identities. These terms, reflecting sexual bias and misunderstandings, cause women who love women to be perceived in a negative light.

In contrast, a range of new *ying rak ying* self-definition terms have been coined within Internet communities in the past four to five years, and to date generally remain limited to in-group use. These new expressions include:

- **tom one-way** (ทอมวันเวย์): refers to a *tom* who is strictly the sexually active partner (*fai ruk*) with a *dee* partner.
- **tom two-way** (ทอมทูเวย์): refers to a tom who can also allow her *dee* partner to be the sexually active party.
- **les** (เลส): a contraction of *lesbian*, refers to a woman whose feminine expressions or attire do not differ from other women (*phu-ying*) but who prefers women as partners. *Les* do not distinguish between gendered *tom* and *dee* roles in a

relationship, but may distinguish between active, *les king* (เลสคิง), and passive, *les queen* (เลสควีน) roles when it comes to sex.

Many more terms also exist. Their use depends on the people or the particular *ying rak ying* community that introduced them, and whether or not they have since gained popularity. However, they all reflect sexual roles as a criterion of self-definition, avoiding the ambiguity that the words *tom*, *dee*, and *les* leave in terms of sexuality, and underlining one's sexual role in order to facilitate relationship building and in-group communication.

The words *kathoey*, *tom*, *dee*, *ying rak ying*, and the newer terms summarized above reflect the complex and diverse aspects of gender and sexuality when constructing the identities of women who love women. They also reflect the difficulty of describing all women who love women with a single term.

The term *ying rak ying* was used in the past to emphasize equality between all groups of women who love women, but today it leads some people to overlook the diverse gender and sexual identities of this group of women. Furthermore, the emphasis it puts on love and romance may lead to female sexual identities being ignored, which would undermine an important aspect in creating understanding and acceptance for *ying rak ying*. While the introduction of the term *ying rak ying* was an attempt to challenge the thinking behind the binary divisions of female same-sex relationship gender roles into *toms* and *dees*, on the one hand, and sexual roles into active and passive parties, on the other hand, it cannot be denied that many women who love women still retain this framework of binary gender and sexual roles. Perhaps same-sex relationships do not differ all that much from heterosexual ones, in that in both relationship types beliefs related to men and women's roles are applied in interactions, and both heterosexual and homosexual types of relationships suffer equally from these divisions.

Whatever women who love women call themselves, or are called by others, Thai society does not give credence to their identities and continues to view their relationships as mere play or as temporary. This affects the health of *ying rak ying* in many ways, whether in terms of mental health (stress caused by non-acceptance, oppression, and fear of being perceived as abnormal) or in the choice of whether or not to use sexual health services. It is still difficult for *ying rak ying* to talk openly about their sexual health problems with health service providers, since they are afraid that they might be seen as engaging in sexually deviant behavior. These problems may leave women who love women stressed and their eventual sexual health problems unattended to.

The above examples reflect how Thai society accepts and supports only one type of sexuality, namely, that involving heterosexual relationships for the purpose of producing offspring. This leads to discrimination against and inadequate health services for those with other sexual identities. Hence, the creation of unbiased understandings should be the beginning of true understanding and acceptance of diversity, which can pave the way for a society that has truly appropriate health services for people of all gender identities and sexualities.

13 *CHAI RAK CHAI* (ชายรักชาย): MEN WHO LOVE MEN

Sulaiporn Chonwilai

The Right to Love, the Right to an Identity

Like the term *ying rak ying*, *chai rak chai* (ชายรักชาย), "men who love men," is a neologism created by combining easily understood Thai words. *Chai rak chai* means a man who likes or loves men and has sex with them. The expression *chai rak chai* was born together with the term *ying rak ying*, and they have been used together for some twenty years by NGOs working on the rights of homosexuals. The first organization to use the word was Anjaree, which was also the first organization to work on the rights of *ying rak ying*. Using the term *chai rak chai* has the same purpose as using the term *ying rak ying*, namely, to focus on a person's sexual identity in terms of emotions, love, and sexual orientation, rather than on sexual behavior alone, which in this case involves men.

In the past, Thai society did not clearly distinguish between gender (*phet-phawa*), i.e., being a man, woman, or *kathoey*, and sexuality (*phet-withi*), i.e., preference for the opposite sex, one's own sex, or both. Besides *kathoey*, which collectively referred to females or males with gender expressions or characteristics opposite to their biological sex, the emergence of words referring specifically to gender (determined by which sex [*phet*] a person's external characteristics match) or sexuality (what kind of sexual lifestyle [*withi-chiwit thang-phet*] one has) can be considered a new phenomenon. It is, therefore, not surprising that most Thais still cannot distinguish between men who prefer other men as their partners but do not cross-dress or want to be women, and transgender *kathoeys* or *sao praphet sorng*.

In 1997 and 1998, the Anjaree NGO and its allies lobbied against the decision of the Rajabhat Institute not to accept what they called "sexually deviant" (*bukkhon thi biang-ben thang-phet*) students. People who love the same sex (*khon rak phet diao-kan* คนรักเพศเดียวกัน) became a widely discussed topic at this time and Thai people gained familiarity with the terms *chai rak chai* and *ying rak ying*. The term *chai rak chai* has continued to be used in advocacy work focusing on rights, equality, and HIV/AIDS.

During the past five to six years, the term MSM (เอ็มเอสเอ็ม), the acronym for "men who have sex with men" (*chai thi mi phet-samphan kap chai* ชายที่มีเพศสัมพันธ์ กับชาย), used in the Western epidemiological study of HIV/AIDS, has also been used to refer to persons whose behavior puts them at risk of contracting HIV. This expression has been coined because a number of men who have sex with men do not consider themselves as homosexual, e.g., some male sex workers. The definition of a person as MSM reflects an identity created by sexual activities between males without reference to either their gender (or lack of it) or their sexuality. That is to say, the definition fails to acknowledge whether the men involved cross-dress, exhibit cross-gender behaviors, and/or desire a sex change (gender references) or whether they are heterosexual, homosexual, or bisexual (sexuality references).

Chai rak chai is often used collectively for those with a *gay* (เกย์) sexuality and for those with a *kathoey* gender. This is due to a general failure to distinguish between gender and sexuality within Thai society, and as a result of the influence of epidemiological perspectives on the risk behaviors of MSM. However, it is now increasingly understood that *chai rak chai* denotes a man who has a homosexual sexuality, who does not wish to cross-dress, does not express cross-gender behaviors, and does not desire a sex change.

Some men who love men from lower-class backgrounds are not interested in this term's history or political implications but prefer to consider themselves as *chai rak chai* rather than as *gay*, as they feel *chai rak chai* is more contemporary. For them, the term does not smack of sexual deviance and communicates an aspirational middle-class status, as this expression is mostly used among middle-class people.

Neither MSM nor *chai rak chai* are well-known terms among the general public. Activists for the rights of men who love men seem to use both the expressions *chai rak chai* and *gay*, depending on the aims of their organization and the task at hand. *Chai rak chai* tends to be used instead of *gay* in advocacy work for rights, including the right to have this identity, and in lobbying for social equality. It is a more academic and formal term than *gay*, which is used both among the in-group and with outsiders. In this line of work, transgender *sao praphet sorng* tend to be distinguished as a separate group, since the discrimination each group faces and the demands they each have differ somewhat. However, when campaigning on sexual health, both groups tend to be referred to as *MSM*, since both face sexual health issues related to having sex with members of their own sex. Those responsible for arranging sexual health services tend to group both together, or at most, distinguish between those who have had sex reassignment surgery and those who have not, despite the fact that acknowledging their distinctive gender identities and sexualities is essential for understanding the sexual health issues people in each group face.

From Behavior to Identity

Although *chai rak chai* and other related same-sex identity words, such as *gay*, *tom*, *dee*, and *ying rak ying* are quite new, Thai society long ago gave recognition to sex between men, calling it in the past *len sawat* (เล่นสวาท), "to play [at] love." Many men of the royal court and also monks were known to engage in this sexual practice. Although *len sawat* was seen as inappropriate and strange behavior, no one was ever sentenced to death for it, unlike in many other countries. In addition to the behavioral term *len sawat* and the old identity term *kathoey*, many more Thai words refer to men who have sex with men. Generally, they are or were used by outsiders and convey derogatory connotations. Examples include:

lakkaphet (ลักเพศ): a transvestite (lit. "to steal [another's] sex")

chai rak-ruam-phet (ชายรักร่วมเพศ): a homosexual man (lit. a "man who loves intercourse")

at thua dam (อัดถั่วดำ): anal sex between men (lit. "to stuff black beans") (see chapter 19)

tui (ตุ๋ย): to force another man to have anal sex; sodomize (see chapter 19)

phu-chai na ya (ผู้ชายนะยะ): a "*na ya* man," *na ya* being a feminine particle used by some women and *kathoeys*

mai pa diao-kan (ไม้ป่าเดียวกัน): an old expression for male-male sex (lit. "trees in/from the same forest")

ee aep (อีแอบ): "damned closet case"

tut (ตุ๊ด): "faggot"

phu-chai si-muang (ผู้ชายสีม่วง): "violet man," violet being the "queer" color of Thailand

phu-chai dork mai (ผู้ชายดอกไม้): "flower man"

Even the English loan word *gay*, which today is widely used, had quite a negative connotation forty years ago when it was first introduced in Thailand. Back then, few dared self-identify as *gay* in public.

Both the medical field and the media have played important roles in creating new words and explaining same-sex sexual behaviors and identities. *Lakkaphet* is an example of a word used by medical doctors. An old term, it was redefined in the 1960s to mean persons with male genitalia and a woman's mind, based on the belief that one was dealing with a mental rather than physical abnormality.[1] Used as a mental illness category, *lakkaphet* was also linked to the concept of *rak-ruam-phet*, "homosexuality," which was seen as a sexual or mental disorder by Thai psychiatrists, who explained that it was caused by family pressures and could be treated and cured with medical advice. *At thua dam* and *tui* (see chapter 19), on the other hand, are examples of terms created and popularized by newspapers.

The origin of the word *gay* (เกย์) in the Thai language also reflects media influence in the creation of new terms and in shaping the meaning of existing ones. Much of wider Thai society became familiar with the term *gay* in 1965, when Darrell Berrigan, editor of the *Bangkok World* newspaper, was murdered by a male sex worker.[2] Since he was a well-known person in Thai high society, newspapers grabbed the story when they learned that he had liked to have sex with *kathoeys* and young men. The incident also made the police much more interested in these groups. Back then, *gay* was a new word, and revealed a new sexuality in which men had sex with each other but without either party cross-dressing or being a *kathoey*. The word *gay* was first used for male sex workers providing services for foreigners, and both *gays* and *kathoeys* were seen as socially dangerous. This, together with the idea taken from older Western psychology that homosexuality is a mental abnormality or a type of sexual deviance, made the word *gay* very negatively laden in that era.

The negative image of the word *gay*, used together with the psychological term *rak-ruam-phet*, "homosexuality," was further entrenched in 1984, when Thai society discovered that its first HIV-positive person was a man who had had sex with men. Thai society had even more contempt for *gays*, conceptualized as *rak-*

ruam-phet chai or "male homosexuals," after beginning to see them as a risk group for spreading HIV/AIDS, an idea based on the perception that they changed their partners often and regularly bought or sold sex. Amid this oppression and lack of societal acceptance, middle-class *gays* turned to *gay*-specific entertainment venues to make contacts and to express their identities. In the 1980s, commercial Thai *gay* magazines appeared, making *gays* more visible. However, most were still closeted, and a term was invented to refer to them, namely, *aep jit* (แอบจิต), "a sneaking/hiding mind." This term is said to have come from the stage play *Chan phu-chai na ya* (ฉันผู้ชายนะยะ), "I'm a Man, Darling," which was first staged in 1986. Adapted from the American gay play "The Boys in the Band," the play was written by Dr. Seri Wongmontha, one of the first Thais to come out as *gay*. Referring to closeted *gays*, *aep jit* is sometimes turned into the humorous and confrontational *ee aep*. Its opposite is *sawang jit* (สว่างจิต), a "brightly lit mind," or, in other words, an openly *gay* person. *Salua jit* (สลัวจิต), a "dimly lit mind," refers to a person who unsuccessfully attempts to hide the fact that he is *gay*. Well-known columnist Vitaya Saeng-aroon gives the following account of his own experience of being in the closet due to societal prejudices, such as those portraying *gays* as mentally abnormal or as promiscuous spreaders of HIV:

Back then I had to *aep yu* (แอบอยู่ "live secretly," i.e., be closeted), because I really didn't know there was a way out. The word *gay* felt like, well, really extreme. No way would I let that word slip; I didn't even dare to think it. I only had scary images in my mind. It sounded dirty, dangerous, sinful, terrible, and so on. I swear that I didn't say that word for decades, and I'm sure I didn't even say it while talking in my sleep.[3]

Not only the word *gay*, but also *aep jit* (which can also be used to refer to closeted *ying rak ying* as well as to *gays*) is negatively loaded, as it connotes cheating and hiding one's real identity. It is, therefore, used mostly by others when talking about closeted people. *Aep jit* and, especially, the variant expression *ee aep* are derogatory terms with which homosexuals generally do not wish to be labeled. *Aep* reflects the sensitive issue of coming out. It refers to the extent, how, and to whom (family, close friends, society at large) one is ready to come out to. This largely depends on the perspectives one holds toward society and the attitudes, whether accepting or intolerant, that others have toward oneself. One reason that *aep* has become such a negative, derogatory word is that a number of *gays* have cheated on women and have used marriage to a woman to cover up their sexuality.

This is the backdrop to veteran gay activist Natee Teerarojjanapongs' attempts at promoting the idea of *kunlagay* (กุลเกย์), a wordplay on *kunlasatri*, a "genteel" or "lady-like" woman, to refer to what is called a "good *gay*," which, among other things, means not exploiting women as a means of hiding one's sexuality.

Diverse Sexual Relations, Identities, and Kinds of Love

Gay is an increasingly well-known term in Thailand, more so than *chai rak chai* or *msm*, perhaps because it is short and communicates modernity and cosmopolitanism. It is used both by *gays* and by outsiders, for example, in novels, short stories, and academic texts, as well as in pride parades or HIV/AIDS campaigns. The word *gay* is often further defined by another word following it. For example, among *gays* themselves, these three types are recognized:

> **gay king** (เกย์คิง): means a *gay* who prefers to have sex as the active/insertive party (*fai ruk*) only (as the word "top" denotes in English)

> **gay queen** (เกย์ควีน): means a *gay* who prefers to have sex as the passive, receptive party (*fai rap*) only (as the word "bottom" denotes in English)

> **gay quing** (เกย์ควิง) and **both** (โบ๊ธ): refer to a *gay* who can be either an active or passive party in sex (as the word "versatile" implies in English)

Sometimes it might be inferred from a person's manners and external characteristics whether a man is a *gay king* or *gay queen*. Effeminate *gays* are expected to be *gay queens*; masculine-appearing *gays* are assumed to be *gay kings*. However, external appearance and sexual role do not necessarily correspond. In fact, often a masculine-looking *gay* may prefer to be the receptive party, or a feminine-looking *gay* may prefer to be the active party. Importantly, both external characteristics and the sexual role of *gays* may change at any time.

While one's gender expression and one's sexual identity do not necessarily correspond, the division of *gays* into two polar opposites, *ruk* (รุก), "insertive/active," and *rap* (รับ), "receptive/passive," shows that they are not free of the heterosexual framework of relationships imagined as being between opposite types. This division heavily affects *gay* relationships, since those whose external characteristics or sexuality differ from this frame may not be fully accepted. *Gays* themselves may not see the true diversity of *gay* sexualities. And yet, many do not feel that they need to stick to this rigid framework. One Internet posting asked:

> Have you ever . . . after knowing each other for less than five minutes, have someone ask you if you're a *ruk* or a *rap*. I just recently met someone. When I said I was a *ruk*, he just fled (I suppose he's also a *ruk*). Another guy, I told him I'm a *rap*, and he also walked away (I suppose he's a *rap*). Now, when I met one more guy, I told him I'm a *both*, and he fled (suppose he doesn't like either . . . so what does he like? I don't get it.) If it were you, would you ask? Or would you ask just before sex? And if someone asked you, what would you tell them?[4]

This posting attracted diverse replies. Some thought it was best to ask the other party whether they were *ruk*, *rap*, or *both* straight away to gain that piece of information, whereas others thought it was not necessary. Interestingly, the latter group did not consider clear distinctions between insertive and receptive parties to be important, rather for them the role choice depended on mutual agreement and the temporary preferences between oneself and one's partner at the time of having sex, rather than any permanent preference. The following are a couple of the responses to the above web posting:

- I don't ask and I don't like anyone asking me, either. What you like is important . . . like, and then what . . . whichever way. If you can't reach agreement, just hug each other very tightly. That's another kind of excitement. Or else . . . that excitement will make us do just about anything. Sometimes you might hear . . . "I'm exclusively a *ruk* . . . but I'd like to try to let you take me. Softly, then, I'm afraid it'll hurt, I've never been a *rap*, just this once . . ." Not asking is sometimes beneficial.[5]
- I'm a *ruk*. If I meet a *ruk* and tell him I'm a *ruk*, that's the end of the conversation. . . . You have to study some people to work them out . . . some *ruk* guys see me and like me and change into *rap* for me. Giving and taking, it depends on the two people as to how they'll do it. I'm mostly a *ruk* but have been a *rap* before. But I must really, really like a guy to agree [to be a *rap* for him].[6]

Many *gays* are not as strict about the division of roles as people in general may think. In other words, *gay* gender identities and sexualities are fluid and change according to the context, sometimes also even between being heterosexual and homosexual. However, living their sexual and social lives without any societal acknowledgment of their identities or recognition of their relationships causes them to be seen as changing their sexual partners regularly or as the cause of the spread of HIV. Although present-day Thai society understands the words *gay* and *chai rak chai* better than it did in the past, and although there are more *gay* spaces (on the Internet and in the form of clubs, bars, and saunas), more *gay* media, and more openly *gay* people than before, the public images of *gay* and *chai rak chai* are nevertheless still negative. A clear example is that if an actor is reported to be *gay*, he will usually hurry to deny the news (whether or not it is true or false) because such news is seen as harmful to his reputation. Many actors accused of womanizing have responded that at least it's better to be seen as a womanizer than as *gay*.

Prejudice Not Fully Erased

The prejudice Thai society still has against men who love men is partially due to medical professionals who have not corrected the old misunderstanding that homosexuality is a sexual abnormality, and partially due to the clash between being *chai rak chai* and patriarchal values that valorize masculinity over femininity. According to societal ideals, Thai men are supposed to be strong, leaders of the family and society, and not "sissy" (*kratung-krating* กระตุ้งกระติ้ง). Many men who love men have to marry a woman to hide their homosexuality, to pay back a debt of gratitude to parents who expect their son to find a wife and have children, or for professional advancement and security. Many male sex workers do not define themselves as *chai rak chai*, but are able to have sex with men to meet economic necessities, while perhaps having a girlfriend and having sex with her, too.

The health of *chai rak chai* or *MSM* who cannot be open about their sexualities due to societal non-acceptance is negatively affected by their decisions not to use health services. Even those who dare to be open about their identities with health service providers may face problems when they engage in sexual behaviors that do not match the service provider's stereotypical framework, such as the expectation that an externally feminine *gay* necessarily plays the passive sexual role.

The Thai Ministry of Public Health now has clinics to provide services for *MSM*, regardless of their gender or sexual identities, i.e., *gays*, *kathoeys*, and heterosexual men who have sex with *gays* or *kathoeys* are now all grouped together. This generalized way of thinking might affect the decision making of potential health service users as to whether or not to use the services, to tell the service provider openly about their behaviors, or to reveal their bodies for a medical check-up. These factors, in turn, affect the diagnostic process and might mean the client does not receive the services desired.

Although the term *chai rak chai* was created by a group of sexual rights activists to present a positive picture of men who have emotions, love, and desire towards other men, the term nonetheless overlooks some important aspects of being a homosexual man, namely, lifestyle, sexual behavior, and diverse, fluid sexual identities. Each time the expression *chai rak chai* is used it is very important to consider who uses it and for what purpose, because different groups may interpret it differently. Activists advocating equal rights for homosexuals might use it with an emphasis on *gays* rather than *kathoeys* or *sao praphet sorng*, whose gender and problems differ from those of *gays*. Health service providers may use the term *chai rak chai* in a general sense, lumping together *gays*, *kathoeys*, and *bisexuals* as a group of people who all engage in the risk behavior of having sex with other males.

Whichever point of view one holds, it is undeniable that Thai society still has prejudice against men who love men. In erasing prejudice and misunderstandings, the most important tasks are changing the way of thinking on sexual matters and accepting *chai rak chai* identities as complex (*sap-sorn*), diverse (*lak-lai*), and fluid (*leun-lai*) in terms of gender and sexuality, and thus using the term that each *chai rak chai* person chooses as a self-definition.

14 SOPHENI (โสเภณี): PROSTITUTES

Pimpawun Boonmongkon

An Ancient Profession

The Thai word *sopheni* (โสเภณี) is equivalent to the English term "prostitute," defined as a person who agrees to give sexual services to another person for an agreed remuneration. The term is derived from the Pali word *sophini* (โสภิณี), a "beautiful woman," through an abbreviation of the longer expression *nakhorn sopheni* (นครโสเภณี), a "city beauty," or its synonyms *ying ngam haeng nakhorn* (หญิง งามแห่งนคร) and *ying ngam meuang* (หญิงงามเมือง). It is a term that has long been used to refer to women who sell sexual services. Other terms, such as *khanika* (คณิกา), convey the same meaning. Historically, some parts of the Indian subcontinent had such women to attract wealthy travelers to their cities.

In Thailand, evidence of the use of the word *sopheni* can be traced to the early Ayutthayan era, when it was mentioned as an occupation in the *Characteristics of Husbands and Wives* (Laksana Phua Mia), a law text of King Ramathipbodi I, also known as King U Thong (r. 1351–69 CE), which specified a penalty for marrying *ying nakhorn sopheni* (หญิงนครโสเภณี), "beautiful women of the city."[1] This occupation continued into the Rattanakosin era, as seen in the *Nirat Meuang Klaeng*, a poem composed by Sunthorn Phu, who lived from 1786 to 1855 CE. This poem is based on Sunthorn Phu's travels by boat late at night along the Chao Phraya River, where he heard women singing and announcing a gathering place of such women around the Sampeng market in Bangkok, suggesting a possible clientele of Chinese men. In Sunthorn Phu's era, the occupation was not forbidden, but rather a tax was collected from the prostitutes' earnings. Prostitutes were legal and taxed beginning in the era of Narai the Great (r. 1656–88 CE) up until the early-modern Rattanakosin period.[2] In the era of King Rama IV (r. 1851–68 CE) this was called a "road maintenance tax." This term was apparently used because the state used the funds for the maintenance and improvement of roads in order to meet the needs of an economy expanding as a result of foreign trade and growth of the cities. Previously, taxes were collected by "tax lords" (*jao phasi nai akorn*), but later the state collected these taxes directly. In the Rama V and VI eras, prostitutes were called *ying khom khiao* (หญิงโคมเขียว), "women of the green lantern," due to the green lanterns that sex establishments had to hang outside to signal that the house was a brothel.[3] This expression clearly reflects the state's control over the sale of sexual services during those periods.

In the Thai context, the word *sopheni* is used with a negative, disparaging connotation, explained as being a sexual object, being goods for sale, or being a woman who is the "other" (*pen eun*) of society. On some websites *sopheni* is defined as a man or woman who sells his or her body, sleeping with anyone, hoping for financial gain. This explanation is laced with prejudice, since most sex workers do choose their clients, or at least would like to, if they were not prevented from doing so by their establishments or their own economic necessities.

Many terms exist for female sex workers, including terms of abuse that refer to a woman who has sex with many men and are comparable to the English word "slut," such as:

krari (กระหรี่): "whore"

dork thorng (ดอกทอง): "golden flower" (see chapter 2)

ee tua (อีตัว): *ee* is a particle that occurs in the names of some female animals that usually has a derogatory connotation when used to refer to women; *tua* refers to the body of a person. The expression *ee tua* has a strong derogatory sense.

The following expressions are also used to refer to female sex workers:

nang lom (นางโลม): "comfort lady"

nang bang ngao (นางบังเงา): "lady hiding in the shadows"

nang klang meuang (นางกลางเมือง): "downtown lady," a more recent variant of the old expressions noted above, such as *ying ngam haeng nakhorn* and *ying ngam meuang*

satri bamrer (สตรีบำเรอ): "entertainment lady"

khun-nai rong-raem (คุณนายโรงแรม): "hotel lady"

phu-ying ha kin (ผู้หญิงหากิน): a "working woman"

ee nu (อีหนู): *ee* is the same derogatory feminine particle noted above, while *nu* refers to a young girl

kai (ไก่): a "hen"

From Prostitutes to Jackfruit Ghosts

Another group of words referring to sex workers is based on the place where sexual services are sold, or the type of services provided. For example:

nang-ngam rong-raem (นางงามโรงแรม): a "hotel beauty," refers to hotel-based sex workers.

sao rong-nam-cha (สาวโรงน้ำชา): a "tearoom girl," and *phu-ying yam cha* (ผู้หญิงหยำ ฉ่า), a "drinking tea woman," refer to sex workers based in Chinese tea rooms. *Yam cha* is a Chinese dialect term meaning "to drink tea." In Cantonese it also denotes having a *dim sum* meal.

sao kamphaeng din (สาวกำแพงดิน): a "Kamphaeng Din girl," refers to sex workers based around the Kamphaeng Din area of Chiang Mai city in northern Thailand.

dek wang (เด็กวัง): a "palace kid," refers to a young sex worker based in the streets around the old royal palace area of Bangkok. In Thai, *dek*, "child" or "kid," may refer to someone younger than the speaker and does not necessarily denote someone under the legal age.

sao oke (สาวโอเกะ): a "karaoke girl," and *dek dring* (เด็กดริ้ง), a "drinks kid," refer to workers based at karaoke joints and night clubs, also called "cafes" in Thai, where clients invite them to sit, drink (Thai: *dring*), and chat with them, and may also negotiate sexual services or exchange telephone numbers for the same purpose.

nang-ngam tu krajok (นางงามตู้กระจก): a "glass case beauty," and *phanakngan ap-op-nuat* (พนักงานอาบอบนวด), a "massage parlor worker," refer to young women providing massage, bathing, and also sex to massage parlor customers.

nang thang-thorasap (นางทางโทรศัพท์): a "telephone call girl," refers to sex workers contacted by telephone.

phi khanun (ผีขนุน): a "jackfruit ghost," refers to female or male-to-female transgender *sao praphet sorng* sex workers around the Khlong Lot Canal in the old city of Bangkok, where there are many jackfruit (*khanun*) trees.

phi makham (ผีมะขาม): a "tamarind ghost," similarly refers to female or transgendered sex workers around the Sanam Luang field near Bangkok's Grand Palace, where there are many tamarind (*makham*) trees and where sex workers tend to stand waiting for customers, who come by car or taxi and invite the worker to go with them.

kai sanam luang (ไก่สนามหลวง): a "Sanam Luang chick," has the same meaning as the above.

A large group of female sex workers who work independently without an establishment or an intermediary (*maengda*), or "pimp," are called *aep faeng* (แอบแฝง), "indirect," or *khai issara* (ขายอิสระ), "freelance" sex workers. The word *freelaen*, from the English "freelance," is sometimes also used. This type of sex work results from anti-prostitution laws introduced in 1960 that technically ban the selling of sex in establishments. An important issue from the perspective of sexual health is that freelance sex workers tend to deny being sex workers when interacting with sexual health officials who work on disease prevention and distribute condoms, which makes work on their sexual and reproductive health issues difficult.

Students: "Sideline Girls and Boys"

Nowadays, some students, both women and men, also sell sex, either through an intermediary (e.g., a fellow student, a hotel employee, a taxi driver, or an establishment owner) or by contacting their customers directly through the Internet, by telephone, or from various nightspots. Such persons are called *nakseuksa sao sideline* (นักศึกษาสาวไซต์ไลน์), "sideline girl students," *num sideline* (หนุ่ม ไซต์ไลน์), "sideline boys," or the gender-neutral *dek sideline* (เด็กไซต์ไลน์), "sideline kids," all expressions derived from the English word "sideline," which refers to a part-time job. Waiters and waitresses, bartenders, hotel maids, and young women standing on the street in big tourist locations such as Chiang Mai in the north and Hat Yai in the south also sometimes sell sex in addition to their primary occupations.

"Kids Selling Ass," "Kids Selling Beans," "Sucker Kids": Terms for Male Sex Workers

Phu-chai khai nam (ผู้ชายขายน้ำ), a "man selling water," *phu-chai khai tua* (ผู้ชายขายตัว), a "man selling his body," and *phu-chai pai leuang* (ผู้ชายป้ายเหลือง), a "yellow sign man" are all terms used for male sex workers. Customers range from young and middle-aged women to men who prefer sex with men. Many other specific terms also exist for male sex workers. For example, the following refer to male sex workers by the type of sex provided (anal, oral, etc.): *dek khai nam* (เด็กขายน้ำ), a "kid selling water," *dek khai tut* (เด็กขายตูด), a "kid selling his ass," *dek khai thua* (เด็กขายถั่ว), a "kid selling beans," and *dek mok* (เด็กโม๊ก), an "oral (sex) kid." *Nam* ("water") in *dek khai nam* is thought to refer to semen and perhaps is an abbreviation of *nam kam* (น้ำกาม), "sexual fluids." *Thua* ("beans") in *dek khai thua* refers to *thua dam*, i.e., "black beans," a slang term referring to anal sex between men, while *mok* in *dek mok* comes from the English word "to smoke," which is used to refer to oral sex.

Customers: A Diversity of Types

Sex workers' customers are diverse, and so are the terms used for them. For example: *pa* (ป๋า), "daddy" or "granddad," *pa kae* (ป๋าแก่), "old daddy" or "old grandpa," *pa som* (ป๋าส้ม), "orange daddy" (which compares a customer who has come to the sex worker by chance to an orange that has just fallen from a tree), and *pa ben* (ป๋าเบ็นซ์), "Benz daddy," i.e., a rich customer driving an expensive car, such as a Mercedes Benz, all refer to elderly and/or affluent customers. *Pa* is the Teochew Chinese word for "grandfather."

Transgendered sex workers have their own terms for customers, particularly those with strange kinds of sexual behavior, e.g., *khi thut* (ขี้ทูต), a "leper," *khaek ngi-ngao* (แขกงี่เง่า), a "stupid customer," *khaek chorp hai cho* (แขกชอบให้โชว์), an "exhibitionist customer," *khaek rok-jit* (แขกโรคจิต), a "psycho customer," and *khaek kin ngu* (แขกกินงู), a "customer who eats snake," i.e., a customer who likes to perform fellatio on a transgendered sex worker who has not had a sex change operation and has a penis. *Khaek norng ni* (แขกน้องนี) refers to a customer of a female sex worker. Here *ni* is an abbreviation of *chani* (ชะนี), "gibbon," which is transgender slang for a woman. In the expression *khaek doi* (แขกโดย), *doi* is abbreviated from *doi trong* (โดยตรง), "directly," denoting a customer who directly or specifically prefers transgender sex workers rather than female partners.

Diverse Contexts and Conditions of Sex Work

The diversity of terms referring to sex workers and their clients reflects the extent and diversity of sex work. People of all genders and ages, diverse sexualities, and various occupational and societal backgrounds sell and buy sex. Furthermore, places where sex is sold are not limited to brothels, but can include many locations in people's everyday lives, such as public parks, city communities, restaurants, street sides, and various kinds of drinking venues.

"Women's Diseases": Embarrassing, Repugnant Illnesses

Rok phu-ying (โรคผู้หญิง), "women's diseases," is a collective term for illnesses that medically are known as *rok tit-tor thang-phet-samphan* (โรคติดต่อทางเพศสัมพันธ์), "sexually transmitted diseases," or STDs. There are many such diseases, and their severity varies from life threatening (e.g., syphilis, which nowadays is rare but well-known and often discussed) to those that only cause discomfort (e.g., pubic lice). The term *rok phu-ying* rouses feelings of disgust and embarrassment and stigmatizes the patient. The expression has its origins in symptoms that tend to involve wounds and pus in the genital region and make the genitals look dirty and disgusting. Patients with these diseases tend to be questioned as to whether they engage in (or are outright branded as engaging in) inappropriate forms of sex. In the case of men, they might be asked if they buy sexual services. In the case of wives, they might be asked if they are secretly having sex with others besides their husband. Such patients may be stigmatized as being *samsorn* (สำส่อน), "promiscuous."

Who is That Woman?: The Reality of Power Inequalities

While medical personnel and educated people usually use the expressions *rok tit-tor thang-phet-samphan* or *kamarok* (กามโรค), "sexual diseases," ordinary people still tend to use the term *rok phu-ying*, where the word *phu-ying*, or woman, here has the specific sense of a female sex worker. This is due to the old societal belief that women who sell sex spread infections—a belief which is still strong today. This belief is especially prevalent concerning women who sell sex for a cheap price because they tend to have the least power in negotiating safe sex and getting their customers to use condoms, have to receive customers from every level of society, and do so even when they themselves are ill. Society holds the illusion that expensive sex workers are "safer" because they tend to be young, beautiful, educated, and can choose their customers.

STD patients include women and men, people selling or buying sex, and people not involved in the sex trade at all, e.g., women who are infected by their husbands or lovers. Yet, STDs are still called "women's diseases" in Thailand. Some women have tried to re-label STDs as *rok phu-chai* (โรคผู้ชาย), "men's diseases," but so far without success. The term, therefore, reflects an underlying gender-based bias that regards women, especially those who sell sex, as disease spreaders but the men who visit sex workers as comparatively blameless.

The Neglected Scapegoat

Men who buy sex but who neglect to take precautions against contracting STDs can infect women as a result. But, once infected, these women might then avoid getting treatment, especially at STD clinics, because such clinics are considered to cater only to sex workers.[4] Female sex workers, on the other hand, are pressured to take full responsibility for STD/HIV prevention (e.g., in the "100 Percent Condom Use Project"), though it is well known that they lack power to negotiate STD/HIV prevention measures. It is thus not surprising that the number of direct sex workers decreases each year but the number of indirect ones increases.

Terminology Reflects Moralistic Viewpoints

Many terms, such as *sopheni, krari, dork thorng,* and *ee tua* have negative connotations and ascribe lower value, immorality, promiscuity, danger, and association with STDs to the person so labeled. Female sex workers are also blamed for destroying the family institution and being a risk group for HIV/AIDS. Public health officials have tried to introduce softer-sounding terms like *ying P.* (หญิงพี), "P. woman" (P. here stands for the English word "prostitute"), and *khun so* (คุณโส), where *so* is an abbreviated form of *sopheni* and *khun* is a respectful term of address used before personal names. NGOs such as the Empower Foundation have suggested the term *phanak-ngan borikan* (พนักงานบริการ), "service worker," to refer to sex workers. Despite these efforts to change perceptions, people in many contexts still view sex workers from the old, moralistic point of view.

Most women, men, and transgendered people do not have STDs upon first becoming sex workers, but many are infected by their customers. Hence, it is the customers who are the disease spreaders. There is a great necessity to eradicate misconceptions among those providing sexual health services and to instill more respect for the dignity of sex workers. The perception that sex workers are not good people and do not deserve assistance also contributes to discrimination in the medical services they receive.

Elementary Sex Education, Practical Section (For Men Only)

Kheun khru (ขึ้นครู), "to approach/go up to the teacher," is a ceremony in which students pay their respects to a teacher. These ceremonies are undertaken in a wide range of contexts before undertaking further studies or putting the knowledge gained into practice. For example, Thai boxers perform a *kheun khru* ceremony to honor their boxing instructors. The term is also used metaphorically to refer to the first time a man has sex, often as part of an initiation into a group of older men, whereby the junior member is forced to get drunk and to visit a sex worker, who becomes his first "teacher" in sex. With changing patterns in sex work, *kheun khru* might now be performed by a masseuse, or even a girlfriend, rather than a brothel-based sex worker. The term reflects Thai sexual culture, which legitimizes premarital sexual experiences for men but not for women, for whom the term is not used. The term might also be used to cover the embarrassment that clients of sex workers may feel.

Implications for Sexual Health Promotion

The majority of customers of sex workers are married men, or those with regular partners, and come from a wide range of occupational and social class backgrounds. They play a part in the spread of STDs and HIV to other groups in society. Men should thus be seen as the main target group for disease prevention, and should be provided with condoms and education on condom use, rather than focusing primarily on female sex workers. As terms like *pa som*, "orange daddy," and *pa ben*, "Benz daddy," reflect, many customers have the economic power to buy sex (with or without a condom), implying that the sex worker is often not in the position to negotiate condom use.

In disease prevention and the provision of sexual health-related services, service providers need to be aware of the diversity of sex work. This includes awareness of the type or place of sex work, the sexual identity of the sex worker and the client, the type of client, the context and conditions of the sexual life of the sex worker, and the meanings given to various kinds of partners. Sex workers should be provided with resources for engaging in safe sex and for knowing their rights in accessing sexual or reproductive health services. Service providers should offer services based on the diverse experiences of sex workers themselves, seeing sex workers as sources of knowledge, as experienced and resourceful people. However, the most important thing is to deconstruct misconceptions among service providers and thus allow them to base their work with sex workers on human rights and health rights perspectives.

PART 4

SEXUAL PRACTICES AND NEW TYPES OF SEXUAL RELATIONSHIPS

15 *AO KAN* (เอากัน): TO HAVE SEX

Ronnapoom Samakkeekarom

Ao kan . . . Just a Matter of Having Sex?

Ao (เอา) normally means "to take," "to receive," "to lead," "to have," or "to want" but in the idiom combined with *kan* (กัน), which indicates "mutual action by two or more parties,"[1] it means "to have sex." As a composite term, *ao kan* means "to have sex with each other" and "to share sexual experiences," implying equality, mutual consent, and activity by both (or all) parties. It is a general term and is not restricted by the gender (*phet-phawa*) of the people who are having sex. Many other terms also denote "to have sex," reflecting factors like the status or type of persons involved, emotions, power relationships, implicit beliefs and prejudices, the time of having sex, or even sex positions. Some of the most common terms and expressions include:

eup (kan) (อึ๊บ[กัน]): is similar to *ao kan* in that it does not connote any gender prejudice that one party loses while the other gains in sex, as in the idiom *dai sia* [see below]. Rather, it is a colloquial, informal term that connotes forceful physical movements in the sex act described. It also has an onomatopoeic element and refers to the sounds made by people having sex.[2]

pi/pi kan (ปี้/ปี้กัน): actually refers to copulation for the purpose of reproduction between birds,[3] but is also widely used to refer to sexual procreation between two human beings and does not cover other types of sex including, for example, anal or oral sex. It has also found its way into the idiom *kin khi pi norn* (กิน ขี้ ปี้ นอน), "to eat, shit, have sex, and sleep," which refers to the basic functions and activities of human life. *Pi* as such tends to be used in describing sex in a naturalistic manner. Both *don eup* (โดนอึ๊บ), "to be *eup*-ed," and *don pi* (โดนปี้), "to be *pi*-ed," imply that the party being *eup*-ed or *pi*-ed is a woman, that women cannot perform sex on men, and that women can only be the receptive party in sex. This is due to societal values that tell women that they should not be interested in sex or express their sexual desires, so as to accord with the *rak nuan sa-nguan tua*, "to be chaste," ideology and *kunlasatri* (กุลสตรี), "ladylike woman," ideal. Both *eup* and *pi* have long been in use.

norn kan (นอนกัน): "to lie/sleep together" and *lap norn* (หลับนอน), "to sleep together," are also used. *Lap norn* is created by switching the usual word order of the expression *norn lap* (นอนหลับ), "to go to sleep," and usually connotes consensual sex between a husband and his wife.

dai sia (ได้เสีย): "gain-lose," *sia tua* (เสียตัว), "to lose one's body," *pert borisut* (เปิด บริสุทธิ์), "to open up purity," and *pert sing* (เปิดซิง), "to open freshness/newness" (*sing* is Chinese for "new" or "fresh"), all reflect sexual inequality because they involve the moralistic judgment that one party—typically the woman or receptive party—"loses" in sex, while the other—typically the man or active party—"gains." The man "gains" (*dai*) experience, ownership over a woman, and/or an increase in his masculinity; while the woman "loses" (*sia*) her honor, purity, and virginity, as in the idiom *sia* (*khwam*)*sao* (เสีย[ความ]สาว), "to lose one's maidenhood." These expressions are typically used in reference to premarital sex among teenagers. Similar to them are *jor khai daeng* (เจาะไข่แดง), "to pierce the egg yolk" and *fan* (ฟัน), "to cut/slash," terms used by men and considered impolite. *Fan*, particularly, is used by teenagers and connotes a man deceiving a woman in order to have sex with her, as in *fan laeo thing* (ฟันแล้วทิ้ง), "to fuck and run." However, youth culture is beginning to change. Some women now *fan* men to gain *taem* (แต้ม), "points," peer group appreciation, and the title *dao* (ดาว), a "star." A young woman exhibiting this kind of sexual behavior can also be called *dek la taem* (เด็กล่าแต้ม), a "point-chasing kid."[4] The behavior itself seems no different from that of men who use sexual matters as a tool for gaining kudos for themselves within their peer group or society at large. Yet society marginalizes youth culture through constant monitoring of youth sexual behavior as well as by refusing to build impartial understanding of sexual matters among youth and by giving no importance to young people's own decisions.

chik thurian (ฉีกทุเรียน): "to peal a durian" makes a comparison between peeling a durian fruit, which has a spiky, hard rind, and is thus difficult to peel and the kind of sex that a man gains with difficulty—whether by cunning or violence.

Thai people of diverse sexualities and genders (*khon thi mi khwam-lak-lai thang-phet*) also engage in a diversity of sexual practices, just as heterosexual, gender-normative men and women do. However, there is generally little public awareness of these types of sex, or they may be seen as abnormal and unnatural. People of diverse sexualities have consequently created their own, unbiased, group-specific terms to avoid being defined or judged with externally imposed terms. Their own terms are often metaphorical, while more educated men who love men tend to use English loanwords. These terms, often colorful, refer to various sex positions and types of sex, reflecting sexual pleasure in ways that expressions of (heterosexual) men and women rarely do (see chapter 19).

For instance, *ti ching* (ตีฉิ่ง), "to beat cymbals," refers to sex between two women. *Ching* are palm-sized, cup-shaped cymbals made of brass and in this expression are compared to women's sex organs. This term is used by outsiders (who find it amusing), but not by women who love women, who feel it ridicules them and portrays them as strange. *Len pheuan* (เล่นเพื่อน), "to play [with] a friend," is another, very old term that refers to a sexual relationship between women, which outsiders see as implying a playful, casual affair, not a permanent relationship. Some upper class women have recently reclaimed the term to avoid direct references to sex between women.

Used in Thai, the English loanword "sex," pronounced *sek*, refers exclusively to "sexual intercourse" (*phet-samphan* เพศสัมพันธ์). *Mi sek* (มีเซ็กส์), "to have sex," has a formal, academic feeling, and tends to be used by educated, wealthy middle-class people, or by teenagers.

Sangwat (สังวาส) is a Sanskrit-derived loan word used in literary works that portray ancient times. It is still used by writers and the elderly. As a part of compound terms like *sep sangwat* (เสพสังวาส), "to have sexual intercourse," it is more contemporary than when used alone. The often-used *sep som* (เสพสม), "to have sex," has a similar sense. It is derived from the name of a popular newspaper sex advice column, Sep som bor mi som (เสพสมบ่มิสม) (To Have Sex But No Satisfaction), in the *Daily News*, which inspired similar columns in other newspapers that adopted the term.

Praweni (ประเวณี), a Pali-Sanskrit loan word, and *mi phet-samphan* (มีเพศสัมพันธ์), "to have sexual relations," are formal, academic, written terms typically used in public settings.

Yet (เย็ด), "to fuck," an original Thai word, has fallen out of general use, with the exception of men who love men (*chai rak chai*) who still use it, or the variant *ye* as a softer form. However, *yet* is still widely used as an invective or expletive, in much the same way as "fuck" in English, or when referring to sex in a disdainful way.

Objectives and Value of Sex

In Thai society it is often said that sex between a man and a woman should be the result of love and should aim at procreation as well as sexual pleasure. In mainstream society, only vaginal penetration by a penis tends to be seen as having sex, with climaxes achieved as a result of manual stimulation likely to be seen as mere foreplay or as parts of the sex act.

People of other genders and sexualities practice various types of sex. Because these types of sex do not aim at reproduction, their purpose is more explicitly related to feelings, attachment, and the expression of love or lust. For the same reason, they are also more diverse, as are ways of communicating about sexual pleasure between partners, than their equivalents between heterosexual, gender-normative men and women.

The Relationship between *Ao Kan* and Virginity

People of all genders (*phet*) and in all eras have avoided direct references to sex in the Thai language, often using euphemisms instead. This reflects the perception of sex as a private and embarrassing topic, or something between a husband and wife—a matter others are loath to intervene in, even if domestic violence or rape takes place—and even Thai laws did not acknowledge rape within marriage prior to 2007.[5] Thai society still does not accept sex, especially non-procreative sex, as a natural part of human life. This is seen in an oft-cited verse from the classic *Khun Chang Khun Phaen*, "One dies from a lack of rice, not from a lack of [sexual] charm." Those who reveal their desire for sexual pleasure, especially if they are women, tend to be gossiped about by mainstream society.

Thai society monitors women's sexual activities more than those of men, linking them to virginity and women's perceived value. Even a single penetration of the vagina by a penis, whether consensual or compelled, at whichever age, makes a woman lose her maidenhood (*sun-sia khwam-sao*), and hence value in the eyes of society. However, women tend to wonder if anal or oral penetration, or penetration of the vagina by something other than the penis, makes them lose their purity.

A woman's virginity may have been as valuable as her life in the past and is still given much importance (see chapter 2). The societal linkage between a woman's hymen and her purity has led many women who have sex before marriage to believe that since they have already lost their purity, they might as well enter prostitution or have promiscuous sex.

Ao Kan: Types of Sexual Behavior and Implications for Sexual Health

Thai society still holds that the only legitimate kind of sex is intercourse between a husband (man) and a wife (woman), both of whom must be of what is designated as an appropriate age. Yet people of all ages and tastes have various types of sex in diverse types of relationships, including sex between youth or between people of the same sex, anal or oral sex, sex using sex toys, sex between casual partners (*kik*), and so on. Because such non-mainstream types of sex are seen as being engaged in for pleasure only, they lack societal legitimacy and are considered inappropriate. This poses a sexual health risk for people engaging in them. People are also made to believe that these types of sex lead to STDs and HIV/AIDS, while in reality any type of sex can be risky if no precautions are taken.

Sex among young people is seen as a problem and as the cause of unwanted pregnancies, abortions, and the destruction of morality. However, unprotected or forced sex can lead to unwanted pregnancy and abortions among people of any age. Extramarital sex can pose a risk for STDs and HIV/AIDS, especially when a husband first has unprotected sex with another woman and then subsequently with his wife. This has led to disease transmission in many cases.

When *ao kan* is viewed from a sexual health perspective, it becomes clear that moral standards are not appropriate for judging the value of a given sex act. Instead, each act should be judged based on whether it is safe and consensual and whether it leads to sexual pleasure or not. Those working on sexual health (whether in the public or private sector, in academic institutions, or as activists) should analyze these issues to reveal and overcome sexual prejudices in order to finally reach the goal they are working for.

16 *SET* (เสร็จ): TO ACHIEVE ORGASM

Ronnapoom Samakkeekarom

Set: Orgasm or Sexual Climax

The word *set* (เสร็จ), "to finish," normally refers to the act of completing or achieving, and its formal synonyms are *kan-samret* (การสำเร็จ), "successful completion," and *kan-luluang* (การลุล่วง), "achievement," as well as *jop sin* (จบสิ้น), "to bring to an end." Besides this, *set* also refers to the emotional and sexual fulfillment or climax (*jut sut yort*) achieved in both penetrative and non-penetrative sex, including masturbation, and is similar to the English expression "to come." *Set* is used for the sexual climax in both women and men, but its usage varies on the basis of gender and social class.

Common terms for the male orgasm such as *nam taek* (น้ำแตก), "water/semen breaks out," and (*nam*) *ork* ([น้ำ]ออก), "(fluid/semen) comes out," directly communicate the ejaculation of sperm. *Theung sawan* (ถึงสวรรค์), "to reach heaven," compares the sexual pleasure associated with orgasm with arriving in heaven. The English term "orgasm," as well as the expressions *theung jut sut-yort* (ถึงจุดสุดยอด), "to arrive at the highest point," and *lang* (*asuji*) (หลั่ง[อสุจิ]), "to ejaculate (sperm)," are likely to be used by the educated middle classes or within medical circles. Women typically use *set* and *theung* (*jut sut-yort*) when answering their partner's question about whether or not they've achieved a climax. These terms reflect women's so-called receptive role in sex. Men who love men describe the feeling associated with a sexual climax with the word *fin* (ฟิน), abbreviated from the English word "finish," which, in turn, is a translation of *set*. They also use *taek* (แตก), "(water/semen) breaks out," to refer to ejaculation.[1]

Set is a description of a person gaining happiness and sexual pleasure. Individual, group, and societal experiences and learning are involved in its definition. For example, the feelings a woman has when reaching a climax differ from those of a man. The words used to explain those feelings also differ from those used for men because Thai society permits men to talk with each other about their sexual experiences and learn about sex more so than it does women, who must be married to be permitted such open exchanges and learning.

Set has a broad meaning that varies according to sociocultural factors and differences in individual experience. However, Thai society does not differ from the global community, at large, in that medical knowledge is used to fix the meaning of set with reference to bodily mechanisms. For men, set refers to the stiffening of the body, followed by ejaculation of sperm, which is not like flowing water but rather like spurting, caused by rhythmic contractions of the urethra.[2] In women, a state of sexual gratification will lead to orgasm, with rhythmic contractions of the vagina, together with stiffening of the body and the limbs. Typically, there is no ejaculation of sexual fluids as in men, although sometimes there is, and some women report that ejaculation erupts from the urethra but that the liquid is not urine. Although medical doctors do not yet understand female ejaculation well, they recognize two types of women's orgasms: vaginal orgasm, which results from penetrative intercourse, and clitoral orgasm, which results from stimulation of the clitoris. Many women who are unable to reach a vaginal orgasm can reach a clitoral orgasm.[3]

Medicine explains climaxes with reference to anatomy only, neglecting the importance of feelings and mental factors in achieving sexual satisfaction, as well as the feelings of fulfillment or happiness that can result from sexual activity. An exclusively anatomical understanding of orgasms also leads to high emphasis on always achieving one when having sex. Some men and their sexual partners (whether women or men) are led to focus on the man's orgasm and to neglect the partner's orgasm (whether in terms of anatomy or emotions). Those who do not achieve an orgasm, or reach it too fast, are often said to have an abnormal bodily state or an illness. That this state is called an illness reflects a lack of sensitivity on the part of the medical community regarding diverse experiences and various kinds of sexual pleasure as well as the emotional and mental dimensions of set.

Excessive importance given to achieving an orgasm also makes people neglect the processes and methods that lead to orgasm as important parts of their, and their partner's, sexual pleasure. For example, too little importance may be given to foreplay and other kinds of sexual practices that mutually and safely fulfill the desires of both parties, or on reaching orgasms by using the imagination, various materials, or devices. Much scientific and experiential information today presents fixed, excessively naturalistic ideas on how men and women achieve orgasms.

Sexual feelings in men are said to be easily and rapidly stimulated (the opposite being presumed true for women), and an orgasm is said to occur only once for men during sex and possibly several times for women. Methods to allow a couple to reach a physical orgasm simultaneously are also publicized. These ignore the diversity of human sexuality and the various emotional, mental, and spiritual dimensions that are influenced by society and culture, such as masculinity, femininity, being *gay*, lesbian or transgender, emotional states, stress, and age.

Different Pleasures: Diversity among Genders (*Phet*)

Motion pictures, books, and songs show achieving climax (*theung jut sut-yort*) as a kind of completion for sex or masturbation. Today, we are also aware of various medical discourses that construct "truths" about achieving orgasms, based on male and female anatomy and issues like ease/difficulty, fast/slow, once/several times, ejaculation/no ejaculation, and climax/no climax, as well as the medicalization of (excessively) fast orgasms or of the inability to reach an orgasm. None of these approaches explain the emotional or mental dimensions of climaxes or of sexual pleasure.

An orgasm is seen as an important result (in addition to procreation) of having sex. Especially among men, besides reaching an orgasm, another important component of sexual pleasure or pride is that one's sexual partner also reaches an orgasm. Among men, *gays*, and women who love women, those who play the active role (*fai ruk*) in sex tend to ask their partners during the course of sex: "have you arrived?" (*theung mai*), "did you get it?" (*dai mai*), "have you finished?" (*set mai*), "has [your semen] come out?" (*ork mai*), or "has [your semen] burst out?" (*taek mai*). The man might ask because he cares for his partner's happiness or because he wants to show off his proficiency as a *nak-rak* (นักรัก), "good lover" or "a skilled sex performer," or for both reasons. The latter reflects societal values that honor maleness proven through sexual experience and expertise.

Women, on the other hand, may not be able to answer these questions as easily as they are asked by their partner. This is because of Thai sexual ideologies that control women through the obligation to be a *kunlasatri* (กุลสตรี), "ladylike woman," to *rak nuan sa-nguan tua*, "to be chaste," or through the expectation that women should always be sexually innocent. Women are, therefore, likely to respond to questions about their orgasm (*set*) in the affirmative, regardless of their true feelings at the time, in order to maintain the relationship, to express their responsibility in having sex at that particular time, to maintain the *kunlasatri* ideology, or to represent themselves as sexually innocent (even if they aren't). Women only rarely express their feelings or ask for counsel in public, as illustrated by the example below from a web-board posting:

> I've been having sex with my partner for almost a year. I have never *set*. I'm very worried. My partner, he wonders why I'm like this. Am I not normal? He said it makes him feel sexually incapable. I am very worried. Something's got to be wrong . . . can I have some advice?[4]

Many women believe that all people have equal rights to sexual pleasure, regardless of their gender. Such women believe that achieving orgasm (*set*) is a rights issue that should supersede sociocultural factors that are laden with sexual prejudice. This viewpoint has opened up more space for increasing understanding of women's sexual issues.

Among people of diverse sexualities and genders, reaching a climax and gaining sexual pleasure do not depend solely on anatomical factors, but are also linked to sociocultural perspectives on sexual matters. Thus, many such people feel that their orgasm (*set*) is not just about ejaculation, in the case of *gays* and men who love men, but also involves seeing to their partner's orgasm (*set*), being aware of it, or making it happen, before they reach the anatomically defined *set* (ejaculation) themselves.

Diverse Constructions and Processes of *Set*

Medical discourses construct *set* as a state of sexual normality and not achieving orgasm as an abnormality, a defect, or sexual dysfunction. This is especially true for men, because medicine holds the view that men must have sexual potency, be the insertive/active party, and be skilled in sexual stimulation. If a man cannot have an erection, insert his penis into an orifice, or ejaculate (or ejaculates too quickly) he will be considered inferior in terms of sexual ability. However, a woman who does not reach a climax is perceived as normal because it is considered natural in traditional Thai cultural values that women do not express themselves sexually and are not the party that initiates sex.

These ideas reflect prejudiced representations of men and women and engender unspoken standards in sexual matters between men, women, and people of diverse genders (*phet thi lak-lai*). Most people still hold the misconception that achieving orgasm (*set*) is a necessary component of sex. Yet this depends on many factors. Different genders have different kinds of *set* and different processes leading to them. Society considers middle age and old age to be ridden with problems with regard to achieving a climax. Youth, on the other hand, are viewed as having sexual problems due to the fact that they are still searching for their true sexual identities and, as a result, still lack comprehensive knowledge. Mental and emotional states, such as stress or lack of sexual desire are also involved. So are power relations, in which the woman, or the so-called passive party, may not be able to communicate her willingness, or lack thereof, to have sex. Finally, diverse and fluid sexualities are also important factors, for example, in cases in which a climax is reached by stimulation by a partner or an object, by imagination, by pain, by the duration of having sex, by its intensity, or by the amount of pleasure involved.

In the current era of globalization and neo-liberal capitalism, many kinds of devices, food, drugs, and methods are being invented and produced to help those unable to achieve orgasm. However, such technologies cannot help a great number of people, because traditional ideas are used to judge those using them as sex-obsessed or sex addicts. There are also many couples in which one party, usually the woman or the feminine party, has to fake orgasms to maintain the relationship, being yet one more concrete example of beliefs linked to sexual health, which is still deficient among many groups, especially Thai women.

Implications of *Set* for Sexual Health

There is now more professional and popular interest in *set*, due to changes in the meaning given to sex. Today, the definition of sex as a means of procreation has expanded to include its broader significance in which aspects of sexual pleasure and sexual rights are also involved.

Just as achieving orgasm is assigned various meanings through each individual's unique experiences and through various cultural values, not achieving orgasm might not actually be a disease or abnormality (as often claimed by the medical profession). People working in sexual health should, rather, consider the processes that lead to achieving sexual climax, pay attention to safety and the consensuality of sex as well as the implications of sexual pleasure, and consider achieving orgasm (or not) from a sexual rights perspective.

There are now dedicated public sector sexual health clinics in Thailand for men (including ones for men who love men), but not for women, apart from reproductive health and gynecology clinics. This is a clear example of the greater importance given to men's sexual matters, especially their sexual pleasure, at the expense of women and those who have other gender identities or sexualities. Sexual health clinics for women who love women, or even other groups of women are not available. While the existing MSM clinics operate to provide STD/HIV prevention and treatment, they have yet to incorporate sexual pleasure as a key component of sexual health. Moreover, such clinics are still not accepted or understood in the Thai sociocultural context. This can be seen from the stigmatization of service users as so-called "risk groups" or as people who engage in inappropriate sexual behavior. Staff in these clinics may also harbor hidden prejudices, such as disparaging men who love men as a risk group for HIV/STD transmission, even though any group can be a risk group if they engage in risky behavior.

Achieving orgasm (*set*) is an example where the horizons of sexuality broaden beyond those only involving the mainstream frameworks of man-woman sex, sex within marriage, or sex only for procreation. If people can transcend such frameworks, then the sexual health services that are provided may genuinely meet the issues and needs of all genders and sexualities.

17 *CHUAY TUA-ENG* (ช่วยตัวเอง): TO MASTURBATE

Ronnapoom Samakkeekarom

"Helping Oneself": Creating Sexual Pleasure for Oneself

The expression *chuay tua-eng* (ช่วยตัวเอง), "to help oneself," means to make oneself reach a target of one kind or another, including a sexual one, or in other words, to give oneself sexual pleasure or to masturbate. There are many types of *chuay tua-eng*, such as engaging in it alone, in pairs, or in a group, as well as choosing whether or not to use sexual devices to stimulate arousal.[1] The expression *chuay tua-eng* reflects the meanings embedded within the sexuality system and sexual health in interesting ways. Besides the term *chuay tua-eng*, different subcultures and contexts have different expressions with the same meaning. In medical or academic circles, it is variously called *masturbation*, using the English word, or *samret khwam-khrai duay ton-eng* (สำเร็จความใคร่ด้วยตนเอง), "to satisfy desire by oneself," *bambat khwam-khrai duay ton-eng* (บำบัดความใคร่ด้วยตนเอง), "to treat/relieve desire by oneself," or *attakamakiriya* (อัตกามกิริยา), a Pali term meaning "self-sex-action." All these terms and expressions convey a formal, academic, non-graphic description of masturbation.[2]

Masturbation by men is colloquially called *chak wao* (ชักว่าว), "to fly a kite," comparing the masturbating hand movement with that of pulling the line of a kite. This is the most commonly used everyday term, and is used by all social classes and genders, and in all regions of Thailand. *Pai Sanam Luang* (ไปสนามหลวง), "to go to Sanam Luang," is an idiom used by Bangkokians, which refers to the large open space of the Royal Ploughing Ground of Sanam Luang in front of the Grand Palace, where many people fly actual kites (*chak wao*). *Salai norn* (สไลด์หนอน), "to slide the worm," makes a comparison between a sliding worm and a penis being masturbated. *Norng nang thang ha* (น้องนางทั้ง 5), "all the five young ladies," refers to using all five fingers, here called "young ladies," of a hand to stroke the penis. *Khat jaruat* (ขัดจรวด), "to polish the rocket," is also a metaphor for stroking the penis, usually used by youngsters to avoid speaking too directly or too graphically; it is a sexual subculture term. *Tuk tuk* (ตุ๊กตุ๊ก), the name of Thailand's jerky motor tricycle taxis, refers to the jerking masturbating wrist movement, while *lang na kai* (ล้างหน้าไก่), "washing the chicken's face," means masturbating in the morning when waking up with an erection, and is used more in the countryside than in the cities.

People of diverse genders and sexualities, such as men who love men, have many terms referring to masturbation, such as *stroke*, borrowed from English and usually used on the Internet, and especially on the Camfrog online chat room. *Kratuk moi* (กระตุกหมอย), "to jerk the pubes," compares the jerking hand movement of masturbation to jerking pubic hair (*moi*). *Tam taeng* (ตำแตง), "to pound the cucumber," makes a comparison with making *som tam*, the spicy papaya salad made by pounding (*tam*) the ingredients in a large bowl with a pestle and *tam taeng*, the same type of spicy salad but made with cucumber (*taeng-kwa*) instead of papaya.

Terms referring to masturbation among women are rarer. Examples include *tok bet* (ตกเบ็ด), "setting the fishhook," adapted from *tok pla*, "to fish," and *kiao bet khia* (เกี่ยวเบ็ดเขี่ย), "to reach with a hook," both of which refer to using a finger to touch the clitoris or female sexual organs. Another idiom is *len siao* (เล่นเสียว), "to play thrills."

In Western societies, Christian beliefs and teachings have had a pervasive influence on ways of thinking in all fields. Sexuality has also been interpreted from this point of view, and only sexuality within marriage for procreation was traditionally considered legitimate. Because masturbation means satisfying one's own sexual needs, not in order to procreate and not connected to marriage, in some periods of history it has been considered abnormal, sinful, and wrong. This way of thinking has also influenced Thai views about sexual matters, such as in a sex education manual that states: "to *chuay tua-eng* often can lead to mental abnormality or illness,"[3] or in the following newspaper item:

> Why does my husband satisfy his desire by himself (*samret khwam-khrai duay ton-eng*)? The first thoughts that come to mind are: "Oh, why don't you do it with me? . . . You've got something to hide from me . . . There's something abnormal about me . . . What is it that's not good about me? . . . What do I do to make you dissatisfied? . . . Are you bored with me already? . . . You've been sleeping around and gotten a disease . . . Yikes!"[4]

The 13th World Congress of Sexology, held in Valencia, Spain, in 1997, challenged old ways of thinking on sexual matters and demanded sexual rights, summarized as: "One has the right to satisfy one's sexual needs by oneself in ways that are safe and harmless toward oneself and toward one's health."[5] Views on masturbation based on the perspectives of sexual rights and sexual pleasure are increasingly voiced and disseminated within Thailand by medical doctors and organizations working on gender and sexuality. They usually take the form of replies to questions about sexual problems in various media (e.g., TV, radio, newspapers, the Internet). An example is Dr. Phansak Sukrarerk's explanation of masturbation in his newspaper column:

> It is human nature to have a process of responding to emerging sexual desire. It is one of nature's outlets when sexual arousal emerges. There is a sexual response process. That is, first there must be a stimulus from outside—an image, a taste, a smell, a sound, or touch. When the stimulus has reached the receiver or sense organ in the human body, a response occurs. With all of our five senses—eyes, ears, nose, tongue, and skin—and when the receiver has received the stimulus, it will send a signal to the brain, which will reply with a command as to how to respond. Now, just how do we human beings have a sexual response? The brain will process the kind of response we are to have. Having received the sexually arousing stimulus, there are three kinds of responses, namely: to stop thinking about it (whereby the response stops on its own); *chuay tua-eng* or MASTURBATION [in English capitals in the original] to orgasm (which is a basic and safe kind of response to sexual arousal); and, finally, intercourse. But whether it's intercourse between a man and a man, a man and a woman, or a woman and a woman, or intercourse in ways deviating from normal people, that's another matter altogether.[6]

PATH, an NGO that promotes up-to-date sex education for youth, explains masturbation on its website in these terms:

> *Chuay tua-eng* is one option for dealing with natural sexual feelings and desires, open to all people, both women and men, if we're not yet ready to begin a relationship. It's not abnormal. Many young people are told many incorrect things about *chuay tua-eng*—that it's bad, sinful, makes you short, makes you stupid in your studies, or that *chuay tua-eng* too often makes you mentally ill or sexually impotent, infertile, and so on. These beliefs have an impact on behavior. Many

girls are shy to talk about it, and many boys are worried about what might happen if they do it often, even though it's a way for us to meet our own sexual needs. Whether we do it often or rarely depends on our readiness, our preferences, and our health.[7]

Chuay tua-eng: Unequal Happiness

While Thai society has discourses about *chuay tua-eng* as an option for people of all sexes and ages, in reality the way of thinking about masturbation is constructed and reproduced on the basis of inequality and multiple standards. That is, those whose gender is male and whose sexuality is like a man's are allowed to masturbate without being seen by society as abnormal, because society acknowledges that when a man is sexually aroused, he needs to have an outlet, so men should seek sexual experiences and express themselves sexually. This can be seen from the excerpt below from a "love clinic" website:

> The sex drive in youth is strong. The way out for almost all young people in this world is to satisfy desire by oneself (*samret khwam-khrai duay ton-eng*), or *chuay tua-eng*. If one doesn't relieve oneself sometimes, when one sleeps at night and dreams of women, sperm will spurt out anyway. They call this a "wet dream" (*fan piak*). Wet dreams, which might also be called orgasms (*kan-samret khwam-khrai*), are an automatic reaction, related to the ultimate in sexual pleasure (*jut sut-yort*). In males, they're related to the release of sperm. Orgasm (*samret khwam-khrai*) is a response that one can learn about; people will learn ways of stimulating themselves. Most men learn to reach an orgasm by masturbation (*samret khwam-khrai duay ton-eng*). To reach an orgasm generally is a wish of the male party when he desires to procreate.[8]

But for women, masturbation is seen as unnatural, abnormal, and a thing that should be hidden. It is thought that only single women, widows, women with strong sex drives, women who are not *kunlasatri* (กุลสตรี), "ladylike women," and the like, masturbate, because society believes that good women should not express themselves sexually. For them, sex is tied to their honor and being ladylike (e.g., not having sexual experiences before having a family). Waen, a twenty-seven-year-old corporate employee explained:

Although I'm a woman, I do have needs. But I've never *chuay tua-eng*, because it would feel strange. I don't dare to. I'm afraid to meddle down there—women need to control their emotions, not like men, who need to vent (*rabai ork*) their tension.[9]

One piece of evidence reflecting this inequality in men's and women's access to sexual pleasure through masturbation is that words referring to masturbation by women are limited in number and are neither diverse nor colorful, whereas for men a plethora of terms are in widespread use. New terms emerge and old ones change, but almost all are construed and reproduced with reference to the male sex organs. Men also discuss masturbation more than women or other genders do because society assigns a higher value to men's masturbation, viewing it as being linked to satisfaction of natural sexual needs and the release (*ploi*) of both emotions and sperm. Statistical surveys also show that women actually masturbate less than men, both in Thailand and abroad, due to misunderstandings, feelings of it being inappropriate, guilt, embarrassment, fear, and so on.[10]

Chuay tua-eng: Happiness Enmeshed in Beliefs

While sexual rights and sexual pleasure perspectives are increasingly influential in shaping Thai people's sexual lifestyles, old beliefs and prejudices based on the idea of sex for procreation only are still powerful. The kinds of questions asked by both men and women regarding masturbation reflect sexual values, meanings, and the fact that standards for men and women are radically different. Men's questions tend to reflect the value of being a man, e.g., Does frequent *chuay tua-eng* make one infertile or mentally abnormal? How many times is appropriate? Women, on the other hand, tend to worry about their image and whether they might be stigmatized by society, e.g., Can one *chuay tua-eng* after marriage? Does *chuay tua-eng* make you lose your virginity? I feel guilty every time I *chuay tua-eng*. What should I do? Examples of questions regularly encountered when speaking about *chuay tua-eng* include:

- Doctor, I've got a serious problem. That is, I've helped myself (*chuay tua-eng*) very often since my second year in high school up until today. I'll soon get married, but I'm afraid of having become infertile, not being able to have children. Is this possible?[11]

- Can helping yourself (*chuay tua-eng*) frequently make you mentally abnormal or ill?[12]
- Does helping yourself (*chuay tua-eng*) make you lose your virginity?[13]
- Can you do it after marriage? How much of it or how often should it be done? What should one do if one finds one's child helping himself or herself (*chuay tua-eng*)? I feel guilty every time I *chuay tua-eng*. What should I do?[14]

Only when Thai people manage to deconstruct and reconstruct sexual ideology on the basis of sexual rights—that is, recognizing that all people, of all sexes, ages, and social classes have the right to satisfy their sexual needs in a way they choose, provided it does not harm others or themselves—will old beliefs and inequality regarding *chuay tua-eng* fade away from the sexual system in which they are so deeply embedded.

Viewed from the perspective of sexual health, *chuay tua-eng* is a sexual practice that manifests reliance on imagination for sexual pleasure. It is a way to create sexual pleasure for oneself that people of all ages, sexes, and social classes can use. *Chuay tua-eng* is also a form of safe sex, used as a campaign strategy against unwanted pregnancies, STDs, and AIDS. For women, *chuay tua-eng* has been used as a strategy in sexual politics to create understandings and deconstruct prejudices against the sexuality of women, who are socially restricted from attaining sexual pleasure, in order to build equal access to sexual pleasure for all sexes. It is also a practice for increasing legitimacy and acceptance for women's sexual matters.

18 CHAI PAK (ใช้ปาก): TO HAVE ORAL SEX

Ronnapoom Samakkeekarom

"Using the Mouth": A Variety of Sexual Expressions and Behavior

The newspaper *Nation Weekly* states:

> Using the mouth (*kan-chai pak* การใช้ปาก) or making love with the mouth (*kan-tham rak duay pak* การทำรักด้วยปาก) has been with us since ancient times. It hasn't just become popular recently. It's called "oral sex" [English in original], which means using the mouth and the tongue on a person's sexual organs. Making love (*tham rak*) with the mouth might also be a method of stimulation to initiate other sexual activities.[1]

However, before terms like "oral sex" and *kan-chai pak* were coined, Western medicine described it with terms like "fellatio," i.e., a woman using her mouth on a man's sexual organs, which is more commonly known in English as a "blow job." If a man uses his tongue on a woman's sexual organs, it is medically known as "cunnilingus," and when people use their tongue to stimulate their partner's anus, it is colloquially called "rimming."[2] In Thailand, murals provide ample evidence of oral sex since ancient times.

The first translated terms in Thai for this sexual practice, used in sexological and psychological textbooks, were *otthakam* (โอษฐ์กาม) and *kama-ot* (กามโอษฐ์). Both are literal translations of "oral sex" using Pali/Sanskrit terms and are still sometimes found in academic textbooks. They are also found in Thai translations of the canonical Buddhist scriptures, the *Tripitaka*, which uses these terms to describe a type of *pandaka*, or person considered unsuitable for ordination into the Buddhist monkhood due to engaging in the behavior of performing oral sex on men.[3]

There are many forms of oral sex, depending on the gender of the person performing it and how it is performed. The Thai language reflects this diversity. For example, using the mouth or the tongue on a man's sexual organs is generally referred to with terms such as: *om* (อม), "to suck and hold in the mouth," *dut* (ดูด), "to suck up into the mouth," *kin ngu* (กินงู), "to eat the snake," *kin ai tim* (กินไอติม), "to eat ice cream," or *pao pi* (เป่าปี่), "to play/blow a pipe."

The in-group terminology of men who love men is more colorful and modern, and reflects the fun involved, and needs to be examined and interpreted in order to be better understood. For example, *mok* (โม๊ค) from the English verb "to smoke" corresponds to *dut*, "to suck." The term *karaoke* (คาราโอเกะ) compares oral sex to holding a microphone close to the mouth when singing karaoke. *Thawai bua* (ถวายบัว), "to make a lotus flower offering," and *bua* (บัว), a "lotus," were originally homophonic puns on the Thai pronunciation of the French word *boire*, "to drink." Later this expression diversified, with versions such as *bua riang* (บัวเรียง), *bua pheuan* (บัวเผื่อน), and also the onomatopoeic *buap* (บ๊วบ). *Soi mamuang* (สอยมะม่วง), "to cut the mango," means using one's mouth and tongue to lick the testicles, which Thai women rarely do on men. For licking the anus, the expression *lang tu yen* (ล้างตู้เย็น), "to wash/clean the fridge," is used to refer to cleaning a refrigerator full of food. *Yok sot* (ยกซด), "to raise [a glass/noodle bowl] to drink," refers to raising the anus to let it be licked.[4]

Many more terms are in general use, such as *tham rak thang-pak* (ทำรักทางปาก) and *tham rak duay pak* (ทำรักด้วยปาก), both translated as "making love with the mouth," *dut ai tim* (ดูดไอติม), "to suck up ice cream," and *om kluay* (อมกล้วย), "to suck on the banana." Terms for using the mouth on various parts of a woman's body generally relate to licking or the tongue, such as *lia* (เลีย), "to lick," *long lin* (ลงลิ้น), "to dip the tongue," *chai lin* (ใช้ลิ้น), "to use the tongue," *lia hoi* (เลียหอย), "to lick the shellfish," and *dut hoi* (ดูดหอย), "to suck the shellfish."

Not Just Anybody Dares to Use the Mouth (*chai pak*)

The borrowed English expression "oral sex" was first used in the Thai context by the educated middle classes, who were able to communicate in English and were attempting to sound academic or trying to avoid using overly graphic or direct descriptions such as *kan-chai pak*. Dr. Prawit Phisanbutr, who studied medicine in the United States, wrote:

Foreign textbooks indicate that "oral sex" is a standard kind of sexual position and that highly educated people are particularly fond of it. In Thailand "oral sex" is considered a type of sex seen often in foreign countries.[5]

The majority of people in Thailand do not practice oral sex or, at least, most people don't say they have practiced it. Those practicing it tend to be urban and middle class because they are more open to receiving both information and outside cultural influences than those who think of sexual matters in a traditional way. These traditionalists believe that sex that doesn't take place for procreation or within the family context is abnormal, dirty, and inauspicious. They view it in terms of putting the mouth (which is for eating) in contact with sex organs (which are the source of various secretions and are considered lowly, especially women's sex organs).

Monruedee Laphimon, a researcher and a member of the organizing team of the second workshop on Gender and Sexuality in Thailand and Laos (arranged by the Southeast Asian Consortium in Laos in 2006) recounted that when oral sex was being discussed, a Laotian man began to look revolted and commented, "The smell of cunt. . . . I wanna throw up." He wondered how anyone could engage in oral sex. Quite similar was one young woman's perspective expressed in a letter to a sexual health column in a political weekly: "So disgusting . . . just the thought of me using my mouth on that part of him is revolting. It's bound to be dirty . . . Really, how can anyone put a clean mouth down there?"[6]

However, when middle-class people are open to the idea that sexual pleasure is a part of sexual health and that everyone has a right to it, oral sex is both practiced and talked about more, as seen from the following newspaper items:

- Yes, it's clean. That part of her is really clean. Every time I use my mouth on that part of her, that clean, arousing smell emerges, especially around mid-menstrual cycle. The lubricant that comes out has a smell that's said to attract a sexual partner. Is it called "pheromones?" Just the thought of it makes the day pass quickly, as I'd like to hurry back home to do it for her.
- It's exciting to watch his weapon (*awut*) pulsate in front of me. His is quite big; he's an athlete. And he massages it all the time. But when I start to do it for him, he just forgets everything. Once he got so excited that his sperm spurted out and filled my mouth. It was quite sweet.[7]

A Form of Sexual Pleasure and/or a Tool of Power

Oral sex has a dimension of power inequality between the party using their mouth and the party on whom they use it. In the context of heterosexual relationships, the man is usually the party initiating it, coaxing or forcing the woman into either using her mouth or into allowing him to use his mouth on her each time the couple has sex. This results from the idea that the man should be the party with sexual knowledge, expertise, and initiative, and that the more sexual expertise he has, the more he is admired by society as sexually proficient.

In contrast to this stands the societal expectation that women should be sexually innocent, passive, and receptive. Women are socialized into accepting the idea that they have a responsibility to fulfill the sexual needs of their male partner. Hence, women are unlikely to dare to suggest using the mouth (*kan-chai pak*), and when they do, they can expect to be questioned as to from where or from whom they came to know of such things. Women seen as knowledgeable in sexual matters are looked down on. If they are not sex workers, the perception is that they must have had sex with many men, which will damage their standing and reputation as "good women."

Women subscribing to mainstream sexual ideology tend to consider the sexual organs to be dirty, lowly, and embarrassing, and that women capable of using the mouth (*kan-chai pak*) must be sex workers. Hence, women are generally embarrassed about and unwilling to engage in oral sex. Those who do use the mouth are likely to have been forced into it, either directly or out of necessity to maintain their relationship. Women are, therefore, unlikely to view using the mouth as a preferred type of sex, a technique, or alternative form of sexual pleasure. For women, it generally represents a duty necessary to maintain a relationship, e.g., some women when menstruating do not wish to have vaginal sex but agree to perform oral sex to please their partners.[8] The male sexual power over women is reflected in the following excerpt from a newspaper article:

> I have wanted her to make love (*tham rak*) to me with her mouth ever since we first fell in love, and she does, with happiness and excitement. Every time she does it and then raises her eyes to look at me, it's true happiness. It shows that she really loves me and has never looked down on any part of my body.[9]

However, for men who love men, using the mouth is a form of sex performed in many kinds of situations in a relationship or between those living as a couple.

Both the active/insertive and the passive/receptive parties use their mouths to exchange sexual pleasure. However, those who sell sexual services sometimes have to perform oral sex on their clients even when they do not want to, or don't feel comfortable about it, because the buying party is more powerful.

During the HIV/AIDS epidemic, oral sex was considered a safe option because HIV is not easily transmitted through saliva. Among young people, using the mouth is also one type of sex that does not involve the risk of unwanted pregnancy.

There is some empirical evidence that middle-class Thais are not the only ones increasingly using the mouth in sex. For example, in the experience of Soibun Saithong, a researcher at the Center for Health Policy Studies, Mahidol University, who has conducted research in northeastern Thailand, rural people there also know of and use the English term *oral sex*, partially because they have learnt about more diverse types of sex from porn videos, which have become increasingly accessible with the falling prices of VCD and DVD players.

Means and Types of Sexual Practice that Lead to Sexual Health

Those who view using the mouth as a type of sex for creating sexual pleasure see it as one kind of stimulation to increase sexual arousal. However, some view it as mere foreplay, as evidenced by various cartoons, porn films, columns, and books dedicated to giving advice on sexual problems. Those providing the advice tend to recommend beginning sex with oral stimulation but also imply that oral sex is not what is thought of as real sex (*phet-samphan thae-jing*), for which only penetration qualifies. The materials of a health promotion project by the Holistic Press (1999) provide one such example:

> Oral sex is one way to make a woman have an orgasm. Some women usually don't have orgasms, but many women can have impressive orgasms by simply thinking positively about themselves.[10]

Viewed from the perspective of sexual health, using the mouth is not only one possible, creative way to enjoy sex; it also helps prevent pregnancies and provides an alternative to penetrative sex. This provides an option for those who cannot engage in it, whether due to pregnancy, menstruation, or because they don't like it.

However, using the mouth (*kan-chai pak*) can also pose risks for sexual health, if those engaging in it do not consider the risk of STDs, or lack information, understanding, or access to protective devices, like condoms. As Dr. Prawit Phisanbutr states, "having unprotected oral sex with an infected person can lead to gonorrhea, condyloma, syphilis, herpes, hepatitis, and HIV/AIDS, the latter in the case of having wounds in the mouth."[11] Most importantly, each time a sexual act takes place, it should be ascertained whether it is based on both parties' mutual desires and whether disease prevention measures have been taken.

On the one hand, using the mouth can improve sexual health, but it can also endanger it, depending on the circumstances. To create a health system that promotes sexual health, health services personnel and everyone in society alike must refrain from judging the value of sexual behaviors like *kan-chai pak* on the basis of mere sexual prejudice. Instead, we should consider the safety of and consent to sex, and the right that everyone has to sexual pleasure.

19 *TUI* (ตุ๋ย): TO SODOMIZE

Ronnapoom Samakkeekarom

Tui: Constructing Negative Connotations for Anal Sex

The slang word *tui* (ตุ๋ย) refers to anal sex between men and is widely used in print media. Its first appearance seems to have been in a newspaper headline about a civil servant accused of sexually violating a boy in 1998. Tabloids turned the story into the biggest news item of the time, adopting the nickname of the perpetrator, Tui, as a new term to suggest the use of force, lack of consent, and sexual violence involved in the act, as well as viewing the act as a crime.[1] *Tui* is often used to describe relationships between males where one party has more power than the other, e.g., an adult and a child, a teacher and a student, a monk and a novice, an uncle and a nephew, or a senior student and a junior one. Some of the various newspaper headlines that have used the term include:

- American teacher caught for *tui*-ing a kid after hiding out in Thailand for five years.[2]
- *Tui* MP acquitted, not involved with boy victim—Pramot secretly marries a Phuket millionairess.[3]
- *Tui/thua dam* teacher goes back on his word—denies all charges.[4]

Before *tui* was coined and popularized by the media, especially by newspapers, *thua dam* (ถั่วดำ), "black beans," and *at thua dam* (อัดถั่วดำ), "to stuff black beans," were already popular terms to describe Thailand's culture of men who love men. Like *tui*, these terms came from the nickname of a man who had sex with boys, as reported by the *Sri Krung* newspaper on June 30, 1935:

On the eighteenth of this month at 18:00 hours, Pol. Lt. Sawaeng Thepanawin, inspector at Porm Prap police station, arrested Mr. Karun Phasuk, or Mr. Thua Dam, of Trok Thua Ngork Subdistrict, Porm Prap District, and brought him in for questioning at Porm Prap. The reason for the arrest of Mr. Karun, or Thua Dam, was that Pol. Lt. Sawaeng had seen that in the shophouse that Mr. Thua Dam was renting, there were numerous boys aged ten to sixteen. Pol. Lt. Sawaeng thus suspected that these boys might be behaving in a perverse way. Pol. Lt. Sawaeng investigated the matter for two to three days and discovered that Mr. Thua Dam is a person who has no wife and who had invited boys to the cinema, had bought toys for them, had given them sweets to eat, and then brought them to his room, where he first satisfied these boys' lust, and then arranged these boys to satisfy his own lust and that of his guests. Those who came to the room had to pay Mr. Thua Dam as if paying for the services of women.[5]

Ever since the press publicized this case, *thua dam* has been used to describe anal sex between men, being a more neutral term than *tui*. *At thua dam*, "to stuff black beans," is cruder than *thua dam* alone. Both *tui* and *thua dam* reflect the history of the coining and reproduction of words and meanings related to anal sex between men by the media, especially newspapers.

Tui is a stigmatizing, negative representation, reflecting prejudice against the sexualities of men who love men. The imagery portrayed by this word makes society perceive men who love men as people who have anal sex and commit sexual violence against men. Obviously, people of all genders can commit sexual violence, but the historical lack of social space, together with the lack of alternative labels for the sexual behavior of men who love men, have made *tui*, along with the sexual violence it connotes, symbols of this group. Most notably, the terms *tui* and *thua dam* were created and reproduced by outsiders, not by men who love men themselves, who often do not like to use these terms and are not happy about others using them either. The same is true for the expressions *khao pratu lang* (เข้าประตูหลัง), "to enter by the back door," *khao khang lang* (เข้าข้างหลัง), "to enter from behind," and *sort sai thang thawan-nak* (สอดใส่ทางทวารหนัก), "to penetrate the anus," all of which are used by outsiders to label male-male sexual behaviors. Also in this category is *fan dap* (ฟันดาบ), "to fence (with swords)," which portrays two penises interacting. When men who love men talk about male-male sex among themselves, they tend to use expressions such as *dai kan* (ได้กัน), "to get each other," *mi sek kan* (มีเซ็กส์กัน), "to have sex with each other," *ao kan* (เอากัน), "have sex" or *ye kan* (เยกัน), "to fuck" (see chapter 15).

Linguistic Practices that Communicate More than Just Sexual Behavior

The term *tui* implies that sex between men is abnormal, violent, or risky in terms of STD transmission. Not only do the implicit attitudes communicated by this term shape societal awareness of men who love men, they also create images that perpetuate sexual prejudice towards these men. Thai society views same-sex love as unnatural and abnormal, perceptions that are entrenched by stereotypical misconceptions of men who love men as having casual sex and changing their partners easily. Coupled with the context of the HIV/AIDS epidemic, men who love men, in general, are considered a major risk group that needs to be subjected to constant monitoring and campaigning. They are referred to with the term *rak-ruam-phet* (รักร่วมเพศ), translatable as either "homosexual" or "loving intercourse," and are seen as promiscuous. All of these phenomena push men who love men to the margins of society. Such perceptions contribute to Thai society's lack of neutral words for describing male-male sexual behaviors and identities and to its use of prejudicial terms such as *tui* instead.

The more society looks disparagingly at and monitors male-male sexual behavior, the greater the influence of negative representations and prejudices, as reflected in these newspaper headlines:

- Vengeful youngster—passes out after drinking, is *tui*-ed by *gay*, runs amok—shoots *gay* in the middle of a market; [*gay*] dies on the spot.[6]
- This is the year of bisexual men (*seua bai*): from the original level-eight *tui* civil servant to a teacher *tui*-ing a whole class of pupils, and a father *tui*-ing his four-year-old son.[7]
- Teacher admits *tui*-ing a child—once heartbroken, now hates women.[8]

These media images and prejudices related to *tui* have been perpetuated through language practices and have created an image of men who love men as being more prone to sexual violence than other groups. Yet, as sexual violence is based on the idea of using power and not respecting the rights of other people to their bodies or their sexual or human rights, people of any gender or sexuality can be perpetrators of sexual violence. People of all genders and sexualities can also become victims of sexual violence in the context of inequality and lack of respect for the rights of others.

The use of the word *tui* by the media has not been all negative, as it has conveyed the truth that victims of sexual violence in Thai culture are those who lack power. This is due to their inability to negotiate and refuse sexual advances or to protect themselves, and involves, namely, children, subordinates, students, and younger relatives; that is, people with less seniority and lower social and economic status than those who victimize them. This has created social awareness of such contexts as possibly leading to sexual violence, and presents challenges to the Thai sociocultural system, in which inequalities still remain.

The Language of Resistance: Implications for Sexual Health

Terms that men who love men create to describe their own sexualities and use among themselves have quite specific meanings. Such terms can emerge, change, and disappear at any time. Unlike the language employed by the mainstream press in Thailand, terms that these men use to communicate with society at large do not connote the use of force or power in sexual relationships but instead refer more neutrally to practices or behaviors, such as *sik* (ซิก) or *siap* (เสียบ), "to penetrate," *o ye* (โอเยห์), from the English "Oh, yeah!" (an exclamation that might be made while having sex), or *ye* (เย), adapted from the Thai word *yet* (เย็ด), "to fuck." Other terms include *do* (โด๊ะ) and *jo* (โจ๊ะ), both of which mean "to fuck," and *nang thian* (นั่งเทียน), "to sit on the candle," which refers to anal sex involving sitting on a man's erect penis. *Kep sabu* (เก็บสบู่), "to pick up the soap," comes from Western motion pictures that portray male prisoners dropping a bar of soap in the shower and bending over to pick it up, and which Thai audiences mistakenly interpret as showing a readiness to have sex. *Yok kha* (ยกขา), "to lift the legs," refers to anal penetration where the receptive party lifts his legs up.[9] The construction of these terms and expressions reflects processes of societal struggle, resistance, and appropriation, and shows the existence of an alternative set of truths regarding male-male sex among sexualities that refuse to succumb to the prejudice carried by the word *tui*. The construction of these truths also communicates that the use, or abuse, of power is not all there is to the sexualities and relationships of men who love men.

Although both middle- and lower-class people use the word *tui* in reference to sexual violence, indecency, or the use of power in male-male sex, the term has also been widely adopted by men who love men, who do not necessarily imply the use of force when using this term.[10] Rather, they use it to describe sexual behaviors that involve following one's sexual preferences and desires, as well as gaining sexual pleasure. Thus, while *tui* is well-known as a word that describes the sexuality of men who love men in a prejudicial and oppressive way, these men have attempted to deconstruct its meaning and present the word as referring to sex that is consensual and enjoyable. The dimensions of safer sex and disease prevention are, nonetheless, absent from these language practices. Hence, those working on sexual health, gender, or sexuality issues should pay more attention to the power of language and the sexual misconceptions that are associated with it in their attempts to create services that are appropriate for all genders and sexualities, and which are free of old, mainstream sexual prejudices.

20 *SWINGING* (สวิงกิ้ง): PARTNER SWAPPING

Ronnapoom Samakkeekarom

Swinging: A Foreign Sexual Practice Adopted in Thailand?

In English, the term "swinging" can mean: "(i) to be fashionable, modern; (ii) animate, lively, active; or (iii) to like to change one's sexual partner often (slang)."[1] In reference to sexual behavior or sexual culture, it denotes the exchange of sexual partners for sexual pleasure without a long-term relationship or love. A person who enjoys swinging is called a "swinger." Those who have sex with other couples in the same room are called "soft swingers," whereas those involved in group-sex are called "hard swingers." While the words "swinging" and "swinger" now are somewhat dated in the English-speaking world, and tend to have resonances of the 1960s sexual revolution, as in "swinging [trendy] London," in Thailand the term *swinging* (สวิงกิ้ง), in the sense of partner swapping, is still very common.

Swinging is thought to have begun as a result of married couples getting bored with their repetitive sex lives, although it might not always be the case of love having been exhausted. While boredom may be what drives some couples to look for something to supplement and enliven their lives together as a couple, even if only for a short while, there are also other reasons for changing one's sexual partner. These might include attempting to increase one's sexual pleasure, or preventing secret affairs, or even trying to increase sexual freedom and equality between men and women. As *swinging* became better known in Thailand, the desire to exchange experiences spread into broader circles, such as among homosexuals, single people, and unmarried young couples.[2]

Swinging women, however, tend to lack negotiating power, as reflected by the use of the expression *kha mia* (ค้าเมีย), "wife trading," used in the 1980s "real-life" book *Game laek khu* (The Partner-Swapping Game) by Phaet Sandot. The book tells the story of a married, employed, middle-class woman who goes to the seaside with her husband and another married couple. The two couples later switch partners and, according to the narrator, have sex following an agreement between the husbands. One time leads to others, and eventually they also switch partners with other couples, as the following excerpt illustrates:

> With this understanding, we practiced it regularly. We soon met two other couples who did the same as us. In so doing, we were strict about birth control, because we didn't want trouble having to wonder who a child's father might be. The news of this husband and wife exchange soon spread far and wide throughout high society. I know that there were four groups who practiced the same as we did—film and drama actors or actresses, gamblers, travelers, and traders. I don't understand how I could stand engaging in those animal-like activities. Sometimes I felt disgusted with myself, but sometimes it was exciting, even when followed by feelings of shame.[3]

Commenting on this case, the author, who is described as a medical doctor named "Dr. (*Phaet*) Sandot," expresses the following opinion:

> This sad kind of behavior is an example of the desire for free sex that is currently spreading in parts of Thai society, although it is not scandalous enough to make it onto the pages of newspapers. I believe this practice is spreading from the obscene societies of those Westerners, because in the early 1920's, after the First World War, sexual desires kept repressed ever since Queen Victoria and the German Kaiser burst out and got free rein, which Western academics called a sexual revolution.[4]

It is noteworthy that while "Dr. Sandot" describes partner swapping as an "obscene" Western influence on Thailand, he remains silent about the long-established and still very widespread Thai "custom" of men taking multiple "minor wives" (*mia noi*), and the act of engaging in prostitution. He also mistakes the "roaring twenties" of the post-World War I period of Western history with the sexual revolution of the 1960s, when "swinging" began in the West.

In Thai society, *swinging* is not a particularly new word or new type of sexual behavior. The word has been in use for over forty years now, first among educated and affluent middle-class people, especially those who had been educated abroad. They brought this type of culture from the West and introduced it into their circles, from where it then spread to other parts of society, such as among single, working people and people of diverse sexualities and genders, such as men who love men.

The word was not previously very well-known within society at large until the mass media began to more frequently report on it. For example, a recent news item stated that *swinging* was among the ten most popular search terms used on the Thai Internet. A few years ago, a girl's guardian reported her as missing and later found a picture of her on a pornographic VCD having intercourse in a *swinging* encounter. Such incidents have led to increased use of Thai terminologies for the practice instead of the borrowed English word "swinging." These new Thai expressions include *kan-laek khu* (การแลกคู่), *kan-laek-plian khu-norn* (การแลกเปลี่ยน คู่นอน), and *kan-salap khu-norn* (การสลับคู่นอน), all three of which mean switching or exchanging sexual partners or *khu-norn*. Some groups use the humorous expression *sek eua-athorn* (เซ็กส์เอื้ออาทร), "charity sex," to playfully refer to the "generous" exchange of sexual pleasure. However, even today, this type of sexual culture is only known and understood among Thailand's urban middle classes.

Sexuality that Conceals Misconceptions

Figures from a National Social and Economic Development Board survey show that Thai teenagers today tend to start having sex earlier than in the past, beginning between the ages of thirteen and fifteen.[5] Teenagers in some parts of Bangkok also like *swinging*, a trend seemingly spreading to larger provinces in almost all parts of the country, and considered a result of imitating behavior seen in others and easily accessible from the media, such as television news reports, pornographic VCDs, and the Internet.

All of the above shows that *swinging* has been an established type of Thai sexuality for some time, contrary to the common perception that it is only a contemporary fad. Internet searches show that there are plenty of groups and communities of people who like *swinging*, such as the Thai Swingers Club, which, according to one website, has more than twenty-eight hundred members. This club's website acts as an information clearinghouse and arranges *swinging* activities for its members. Its ideological justification is that *swinging* is both legal and a personal right.

In 2006, a newspaper reported that a *swingers'* website had been in existence for ten years and acted openly as a point of contact for those who like "group sex" (*sek mu* เซ็กซ์หมู่), who like to exchange sexual partners, or who want to bring their partners to engage in group sex.[6] The website contained images of couples, group sex, and of sexual organs. It welcomed newcomers to *swinging* parties with the following advertising statement: "Join *swinging* for life for 5,000 baht, with parties at 8 p.m. each Friday, lasting until Sunday noon, arranged in three-star hotels."

Members of this website can browse other members' photographs and phone numbers, as well as contact each other directly.[7] The owner of the website, whose username is "Admin," stated that since the site opened in 1998 more than four thousand women and men (in equal proportions) had become members, and that all of Thailand's provinces are represented. Individual membership costs 5,000 baht and a couple's membership went for 7,500 baht, both payable by bank transfer. The registration system was automatic. Members received a four-digit personal code for logging onto the website and could then join the club's various activities, such as the Friday night parties, at no extra cost. One posting on this website read:

Last time, a lot of people came to the party. At the moment, most people who come are foreigners. In the party, we've got food and games, like blindfolding and drawing lots. You can start *swinging* straight away, up to you. But all the people who come are fully into it anyway.[8]

Web-board advertisements also call upon like-minded people to join *swinging* clubs:

We've got a *swinging* club, with couples and single women and men as members. We only *swing* with members. If you're interested in joining, have already tried this, or would like to try, please provide your personal information: if you're a couple or a single person, your age(s), height(s), weight(s), your photo(s). Join by e-mail. New members are welcome. Name/nickname. E-mail/Tel no. *Note*: Your e-mail/tel. no. will only be visible to logged-in members.[9]

Thai traditionalist beliefs that attempt to divide sexualities into right and wrong, without much regard to sexual health or rights, are often used to claim, in a generalized manner, that *swinging* is an abnormal type of sex and implies a betrayal of mainstream Thai sexual culture.

Academics often invited to lecture on societal problems, such as Associate Professor Supatra Suparb of Chulalongkorn University, have explained teenage sexual behavior in terms of loneliness resulting from lack of love and warmth in their families. With families unable to provide this emotional support, teenagers grasp for what they think love and happiness are. They socialize with like-minded friends in the same age bracket, or try to break out of the frame that their parents have set for them, thinking that doing so will be proof of their maturity. According to these authorities, who are often reported in the Thai press and media, this combination of factors gives teenagers the courage to experiment, whether it be with drugs or risky sex, which may then lead to problems like STDs, AIDS, teenage pregnancies, and a reduced value given to virginity and chastity (*rak nuan sa-nguan tua*).[10]

People in the *swinging* circuit, such as Suchart Thanamongkongchai (a.k.a. Ah Kangfu), who was previously a columnist for Thai *Playboy* magazine, look at *swinging* from a different viewpoint than the moralist stance of many social commentators:

As for the issue of looking for *swinging* partners . . . I only serve clients who would just like to change their sexual partner. Usually, they're people who've got sexual problems with their partner and, therefore, have to use my service to find a partner who is facing similar problems. I act as an intermediary, coordinating their meeting. I've done this for dozens of couples already, some of them well-known high society figures. After looking at their case history, or the needs of each couple, I'll look for a suitable couple for them. When they are to meet, I'll tell them their secret code for contacting each other. After that, it's up to them, and if they're interested, they'll switch partners. But if they meet up and don't get along, there's no obligation to go on. Some couples have sex and take a liking to each other, and so they'll meet again without me needing to be an intermediary. It depends on the readiness of both parties. Thai society must understand that the *swinging* culture has been influenced by foreign countries. Anybody can get to know it, because there are many media that publicize these things. As for married couples whose sexual behavior includes *swinging*, or switching partners, we call it a *sex partner control deficit disorder*.[11]

According to this view, underlying the idea of switching partners is usually a desire to maintain a family relationship or to avoid separation. However, it takes a lot of courage for a couple to use such services. It is believed that many more couples are hiding the fact that they have problems but would like to use this kind of service. According to newspaper columnist Wiriya Sathirakul, Suchart

Thanamongkongchai has stated, "I'm certain that there are lots of people with needs like this because, before I was arrested, I received bucketfuls of letters. Some were very famous people."[12]

In explaining *swinging* or practicing it, one should consider the dimensions of sexual health. People should also pay attention to issues of safety, consent, and inviolability of sexual rights, rather than merely judge *swinging* based on old moralistic principles that see it as criminal or abnormal behavior.

Power Relations and Sexual Preferences

Men tend to be the ones who coax their partners into *swinging*, and often it seems that their feelings toward their partners are not negatively affected in any way. Indeed, some say that *swinging* improves their primary sexual relationship, because it adds variety and excitement to it. Some men who have sexual problems with their wives wish that their partners can have sexual pleasure and resort to looking for another sexual partner for their wives. Some gain sexual pleasure by watching their partner have sex with others.[13]

In contrast, the feelings that women have toward *swinging* vary. Some are fully into it, but most feel awkward or compelled to accept when they first encounter the invitation to engage in it. With many women, this feeling of awkwardness persists, yet others begin to enjoy it, and may even initiate it:

> Regarding the issue of *jai taek* (ใจแตก), "moral abandon," it's up to the individual. I wanted to try so I asked my partner to arrange it. First, we looked for couples, but later wanted to try it as a group, so we looked for two or three single men to do a group thing. It was really hot (มันส์ *man*). But I love my partner as much as before; that hasn't changed in any way.[14]

Swinging more often takes place in the context of unequal power between men and women, since men have more power to initiate *swinging*. Unless a woman is equally or more powerful than the man, it will likely be difficult for her to suggest *swinging* to her partner, as this might make him suspicious or lead to her being criticized. Thus, while *swinging* is a non-mainstream way to seek sexual pleasure, it still reflects a continuation of traditional sexual oppression and male dominance.

Types of Sexual Behavior Beneficial for Sexual Health

If *swinging* is explained using traditional moralistic principles such as monogamy, an emphasis on virginity and procreative sex, maintaining chastity (*rak nuan sa-nguan tua*), and so forth, dimensions of sexual equality, pleasure, and health will be neglected as a consequence. However, if *swingers* consider safety (e.g., by protecting themselves against STDs by using condoms) and if *swinging* is based on a mutual desire for it, *swinging* can promote sexual health and be compatible with equal sexual rights. It can be engaged in to increase sexual pleasure, to prevent hidden sexual affairs, or to create freedom and equality between men and women.

Providers of sexual health services should take into account the diversity of sexualities and be sensitive towards this phenomenon. They should view *swinging* as an alternative type of sex that can be safe, if those engaging in it take precautions and do it out of their own free will, and if service providers attempt to build correct understandings rather than assume that *swinging* contradicts Thai cultural norms or is inappropriate. If sexual health service providers continue using prejudice as the basis of their work, the only safe type of *swinging* would probably be that which takes place in the realm of the imagination.[15]

21 *KIK* (กิ๊ก): A CASUAL PARTNER

Monruedee Laphimon

Kik: The Changing Language of Relationships and Thai Sexual Culture in the Twenty-First Century

Among new Thai words related to sexual values no other word is as well-known and remarkable as *kik* (กิ๊ก). Ten years ago it was youth slang and meant "to be cute" (*na-rak* น่ารัก) or "to be adorable" (*na-en-du* น่าเอ็นดู), having been derived from the onomatopoeic word *khik* (คิก), which refers to the sound of a girl's laughter.[1] But nowadays, the definition most people associate with this word is one close to that found in the *Royal Institute Dictionary of New Words*:

> ***kik***: n. a close friend of the opposite sex, possibly within an adulterous (*chu-sao*) relationship, e.g., "You've secretly got a *kik*; watch out for trouble if your *faen* (แฟน boyfriend/girlfriend, partner) finds out." v. to have an adulterous (*chu-sao*) relationship, e.g., "She *kiks* with both a superstar and a singer."[2]

This new meaning was described in detail in a 2004 research study by students in the field of education, entitled *"Kik . . . More Than a Friend But Not a Boyfriend/Girlfriend."*[3] The study, which made the front page in a daily newspaper, reported on values related to love and relationships among youth who like to have several friends of the opposite sex besides their steady boyfriend or girlfriend.[4] Such friends are classified as *kik*. The authors of the study explained that the history of the word is not clear but, in contrast to the view summarized above, they assumed it came from *kuk kik* (กุ๊กกิ๊ก), which refers to shows of affection (*kranung kraning ju-ji-kan* กระหนุงกระหนิง จู๋จี๋กัน). A *kik* is considered more than a friend but not (yet) a boyfriend or girlfriend. One may, perhaps usually, have sex with a *kik*.

Wikipedia offers several possible origins of the word: *kuk kik* (กุ๊กกิ๊ก), said by teenagers to mean going out, spending time together; *click*, which in English slang refers to two people being a good match for each other, i.e., "to click with someone;" or *gig* (also spelled กิ๊ก in Thai), which in English slang means a short-time activity or performance by a band or singer in a pub or club.[5]

In the 2004 study, informants gave various reasons for having *kiks*. Those without a regular partner (*faen*) said that it helped ward off loneliness, was better than being alone, and perhaps the *kik* relationship might one day develop into a partnership. Those with a *faen* said they had *kiks* because they were not sure if their current partner was the right one, or because their partner acted in a boring way. For some, having many *kiks* might be a fashion or a way to express their charm to others. In any case, the important rule when having or being a *kik*—or *kik*-ing with someone—is to make it clear what each person's status is and to accept the rules of being a *kik*, which the study defined as:

- Jealousy is forbidden, but caring for each other is OK.
- Having sex is OK, but neither party "owns" (the heart of) the other.
- There is no right to ask for more than is reasonable.
- The status of a *kik* might change (to become a *faen*), but if it doesn't, no sadness or regret is permitted.
- No sharing of *kiks* between friends.
- If a *kik* wants to have a *faen* and it's not you, no drama is allowed. You must try to accept it and delight in it and later agree on whether or not to continue being *kiks* with each other.
- No need to take care of each other too much, because you're just *kiks*.
- Infinity is the limit for the number of *kiks*; sex, age, and status are not fixed.
- A *kik* is less important than a *faen*.
- A *kik* must know his or her place—if the *faen* finds out, the *kik* must go.[6]

The study's definition of *kik* can be summarized as follows: a *kik* is more than a friend, but is neither a *faen* nor a secret lover (*chu*). Yet, if one party's *faen* finds out, it is expected that the *kik* must go. The report also stated that this relationship type is not completely new and has long been known by different names, such as *dek* (เด็ก), "kid," later *pro* (โปร), and now most recently as *kik*. A study on Thai slang published by the Ministry of Education explains that in this context *dek* means a young woman lover of a man, as in "Yesterday I saw you skip classes to go out with your *dek*."[7] As used here, *pro* probably refers to its second definition in the *Royal Institute Dictionary of New Words*: "v. to like a lot, e.g., 'The boss *pros* this subordinate.'"[8] One media commentator explains that *pro* is an abbreviation of the English word "project" and means "a person one secretly likes," as if that person were a project to be undertaken.[9]

The launch of the Chulalongkorn University study made *kik* a hot topic, to the extent that the word had to be added to new Thai dictionaries.[10] The *Non-Royal Institute Dictionary* by the Matichon publishing group defined the term as "a person who is not a lover (*khu-rak*) but has a relationship like one." This is interesting in that it is not limited to opposite-sex couples. The Thai *Wikipedia* defines *kik* thus:

> ***Kik***, which sometimes means a *date* or *khu-date* (คู่เดท "date partner"), refers to a short-term relationship, different from *faen*, which generally refers to a long-term relationship. *Kik* relationships often have misunderstandings, such as when the two parties do not speak of, or might misunderstand, whether it is a short- or long-term relationship. Currently, the word *kik* refers to the search for friends among teenagers, whether looking for a friend to chat with or to go out with, using the word *kik* instead of *pheuan* (เพื่อน "friend") as a fashionable term.[11]

While there is no certainty about the origins of the word *kik*, it is now popular among people of all genders, sexualities, and ages. Previously, Thai society had a more limited choice of relationship words. On the one hand, there were those that denoted socially acceptable relationships, such as *faen* (แฟน), "boyfriend/girlfriend" or "partner/spouse," *sami* (สามี), "husband," *phanraya* (ภรรยา), "wife," and *khu-rak* (คู่รัก), "partner" or "lover" (N.B.: not a secret lover). On the other hand, there were terms for types of relationships that clash with the Thai sexual value of monogamy, such as: *chu* (ชู้), "secret lover," and *mia noi* (เมียน้อย), "minor wife," as well as words indicating a less serious relationship, such as *khu-khuang* (คู่ควง), *khu-kha* (คู่ขา), and *khu-norn* (คู่นอน), all three of which roughly translate as "sex buddy."

The word *kik* can be said to open up a new viewpoint on the complexity of human relationships. While the relationship type itself is not new in Thailand, the emergence of a cute term that is not predominantly negative for casual sexual relationships is a recent phenomenon that has elicited many attempts to define it. The definitions people give to the term, and the perspectives people have toward this relationship type, vary considerably. Some feel negative about it, seeing the word as synonymous with *chu* ("secret lover"), but others feel the word is cute and helps them to define more clearly their role in their various relationships. Some argue that having a *kik* is a personal right because they have not agreed to be a *faen* with anyone, and if they do have a *faen* then they do not consider having a *kik* as constituting adultery as long as they don't have sex with the *kik*. Another reason for the sudden popularity of the word since 2004 is that the values inherent in having a *kik* have challenged society's ideologies of monogamous marriage and so-called real love, whose adherents became afraid that any challenge to those values would lead to sex among school students, unwanted pregnancies, abortions, and the risk of STDs and HIV/AIDS. The definitions given for the word *kik* in the 2004 Chulalongkorn University research study and the dictionaries cited above reflect Thai ways of thinking about gender and sexuality, relationships between men and women (including number of partners, intensity of relationships, agreements on the nature of relationships), and love as well as sex, whether it be monogamous or not, premarital or marital.

From *Faen* and *Chu* to *Kik*: Inequality and Sexuality

Prior to the emergence of the word *kik*, a limited number of Thai relationship words existed that could be easily categorized into acceptable and unacceptable relationships. A glance at the *Dictionary of the Royal Institute*, 1999 edition, shows that words referring to acceptable relationships usually imply that these are heterosexual and monogamous:

> ***sami, phua*** (ผัว a less elegant term for "husband"): n. a man who is a woman's spouse, a partner of a *phanraya* or *phariya* (ภริยา syn. of *phanraya*, "wife"); owner (Pali, Sanskrit: *swamin*).
>
> ***phanraya, phariya, mia*** (เมีย a less elegant term for "wife"): n. a woman who is a man's spouse, a partner of *sami* (S. *pharya*, P. *phariya*).
>
> ***khu-rak:*** n. a man and a woman bound in love; *khon rak* (คนรัก a "lover").
>
> ***faen*** (coll.): n. a lover, *khu-rak*, *sami*, or *phanraya*.[12]

Of the words referring to relationships outside those accepted within the societal frame, *chu* is an old word found in many expressions. Words like *khu-khuang* and *khu-norn* are not found in dictionaries, but the definition of *khu-kha* as a man and a woman who are lovers (as in, "Everyone knows that you two have been *khu-kha* for a long time") was added to the *Royal Institute Dictionary of New Words* to complement its earlier definition: "stage actors who are a good match for each other."

Of the words listed above, *phua*, "husband," *mia*, "wife," and *chu*, "secret/illicit lover," are probably the oldest ones, all having been used since the era when it was still legal for men to have several wives. Interestingly, the meaning of *chu* is quite complex. It can be used of both men and of women. *Pen chu* (เป็นชู้), "to be a *chu*," refers to a man having sex with a married woman, whereas *mi chu* (มีชู้), "to have a *chu*," refers to a married woman having sex with a man other than her husband. On the surface, these two terms seem equally negatively loaded. However, when looking at them from the mainstream Thai viewpoint on gender and sexuality—which assumes that men have a higher need for sexual outlets than women, and values womanizing men for their sexual charm but restricts women to having sex only within marriage in order to have children—the connotations of these expressions part ways. Thus a woman who "has a *chu*" (*mi chu*) is condemned much more severely than a man who "is a *chu*" (*pen chu*). Although these terms are not directly related to the word *kik*, they are related to Thai sexual relationship ideology. They reflect the fact that mainstream Thai society only acknowledges and accepts heterosexual relationships, and also prefers that they are based on love and lead to a monogamous marriage—the longer the better, and with no premarital sex.

In reality, however, many people do not follow these ideals in their relationships but instead choose a lifestyle based on their own individual desires, such as those who prefer same-sex relationships, those who refuse life as a couple within the framework of marriage, those who enjoy sex without love, and those who want neither marriage nor children.

The emergence of the word *kik* and its explanatory framework has allowed people to use it in interpreting their relationship experiences. Various replies to a 2004 web-board entry, entitled "What does the word *kik* mean?,"[13] reflect alternative Thai perspectives on sex and relationships. These include the view that one can have sex for the sake of sexual pleasure and not merely for having children, as well as the sexual rights perspective on choices and communication between partners. There is also the perspective of applying moral principles in directing relationships, as illustrated in the following responses to the web-board discussion:

- The one you want to sleep with, but not marry. Wanna be my *kik*?[14]
- *Kik* is the representative of infidelity (*khwam-mai-seu-sat*) or the beginning of infidelity.[15]
- *Kik* means having limitless sex, without restraint, without morality . . . oh! I want to have sex![16]

Many people think that *kik* means the same as *chu* and that the word *kik* is simply used to avoid the negative connotations of the word *chu*. However, the 2004 Chulalongkorn University research study concluded that:

A *kik* is not a *chu* because *chu* refers to a *faen* who is not the number-one *faen*, but who is nonetheless accepted and called a *faen*, and there might or might not be sex. Usually, it is accepted that there are both *kik*- and *chu*-type relationships. One might or might not know about one's partner having a *kik*, accept it or not, and may use either the word *kik* or *chu* for this.[17]

Whether or not the two words are synonymous, most people view the word *kik* negatively. Those who have a *kik* explain that it is a matter of understanding and agreement between the parties concerned and a personal right to have or not have one. People of different ages may interpret the word differently, but one should not use one's own viewpoint to judge others. One female commentator observed:

Kik means someone we love or who loves us, nothing is off limits except private matters. If I don't want to tell, you shouldn't want to know. A *kik* is inferior to a *faen*. Not everyone needs one; it depends on whether your *faen* can accept it. If my *faen* had a *kik*, I could accept it, because we study in different faculties and don't have much time for each other. But he doesn't [have a *kik*], anyway. I'm the one who does—ha, ha, ha—and I don't see him blaming me for it (am I selfish?)[18]

The 2004 research study on the *kik* phenomenon stated that men and women have *kiks* to the same extent. However, those who think that men have more believe that it is in men's nature, and assume that men like having *kiks* to show off their power and to have things to talk about with their drinking mates. Those who believe that women have more *kiks* than men think that women don't know how to refuse a man's advances, don't dare to make a choice, are sensitive, and easily fall into the trap of love, or, alternatively, that modern women are confident, dare to express themselves, and like to charm men.

While the emergence of the word *kik* has increased acceptance of love and relationships outside the framework of monogamy, and while it is a general term not limited to one gender or to heterosexual relationships, its usage nonetheless still reflects the double sexual standards of Thai society. Men are advantaged in having opportunities to learn about, or having access to sexual matters, and as the idea of having a *kik* may or may not imply a sexual relationship, men who have several *kik* are not judged the same as women who do the same.

Values Related to *Kik* and Sexual Control Measures

The Chulalongkorn University study brought a wave of criticism and debate on sexual values, and revealed that not only teenagers but also people of different ages and genders had experienced relationships comparable to a *kik* one.

The *kik* phenomenon among teenagers aroused the most anxiety among societal and state bodies, such as educational institutions, families, and the mass media, which were concerned that the values related to having *kik* would destroy what are considered "good," "traditional" beliefs on sexual matters, pose risks in terms of STDs, lead to sex among school-age youth, and increase the number of abortions and other sex-related social problems. From the sexual mainstream viewpoint, a *kik* meant having sex without love outside of marriage, and for short-term sexual pleasure only. Importantly, having a *kik* also challenged views related to the allowable number of sexual partners. From this perspective, *kik* might not, after all, differ from *chu*, which is associated with the word *samsorn* (สำส่อน), "to be promiscuous," as reflected in the following web-board entry:

> Don't you feel strange that we're made to believe that *kik* means *chu*? Teenagers think that a *kik* is an understanding friend on another level, but adults are pushing the sexual implication.[19]

It is not surprising that institutional bodies intent on monitoring the sexual behavior of children and youth interpret teenagers having *kiks* as extreme sexual behavior and a decay of sexual mores, as was seen in reporting by the Ministry of Culture and in the media response to the findings of the 2004 research study.

For people working on sex and gender issues, the *kik* phenomenon demonstrates that relationships linked to gender and sexuality are complex, and that there are many people whose way of thinking on sexuality is outside of mainstream society's framework. The emergence of the word *kik* has opened a space for more people to make their own decisions as to what kind of relationships they should have and with whom. It has allowed them to consider whether they should have sex or not, and under which conditions, and for which reasons. Ultimately, it has offered a space for people to take responsibility for those decisions, in their capacity as individuals with the right to direct their own sexual lifestyles and their reproductive hygiene.

Notes

TRANSLATOR'S NOTES

1. See Royal Institute of Thailand, *Principles of Transcribing Thai Phonetically in Roman Script,* 1999, http://www.royin.go.th/upload/246/FileUpload/416_2157.pdf.

INTRODUCTION TO THAI EDITION

1. Williams, *Keywords.*
2. Wierzbicka, *Understanding Cultures Through Their Key Words.*
3. Bourdieu, *Distinction: A Social Critique.*

INTRODUCTION TO ENGLISH EDITION

1. See, e.g., Van Esterik, "Repositioning Gender, Sexuality, and Power;" Van Esterik, *Materializing Thailand.*
2. Harrison, "Disruption of Female Desire;" Harrison, "Wild Roses."
3. Ojanen, "Sexual/Gender Minorities," 7.
4. See, e.g., Jackson, "Thai Research on Male Homosexuality."
5. Ojanen, "Sexuality/Gender Minorities," 17.
6. Ibid., 30.
7. Harrison and Jackson, *Ambiguous Allure of the West.*
8. Martin et al., *AsiaPacificQueer.*

KEY FINDINGS

1. Fairclough, *Discourse and Social Change.*

CHAPTER 1: SEXUAL MATTERS

1. *Dictionary of the Royal Institute,* 1982 ed., 593.
2. Ibid., 714.
3. Jamnong Thorngprasert, "Phet," in *Phasa Thai khai-khan* [The Thai language unlocked] (Bangkok: Phrae Phitthaya, 1985), 274–75, http://royin.go.th/th/knowledge/detail.php?Search=1&ID=1251 (accessed January 20–25, 2007).
4. "Rup-pan phileuk keuk-keu nai suan Kaoli faeng reuang tai sadeu noi-noi," posted by "dan," http://www.siamha.com/content/data/2/0467.html (accessed November 14, 2006).

5. "Phor. Mor. chao yai ik laeo—reuang tai sadeu phlo ik 1 hua-na suan jangwat luan-lam jap kon luk-norng sao ma pen raem pi," October 2007, http://www.oknation.net/blog/print. php?id=134280 (accessed January 20, 2008).

6. "Reuang tai sadeu kap 'yup phak,'" http://www.kanmuang.org/NT/data/7/0398-1.html (accessed January 20, 2008).

7. "Reuang yang wa thi phu-ying . . . yak tham," posted by "2kung," June 4, 2004, http://www.dcondom.com/00.dclub/club/forum_posts.asp?TID=2628 (accessed January 20, 2008).

8. Post by "Sorn dek," http://www.ruengerotic.com/13/80328_/0/80328 (accessed January 20, 2008).

9. "Reuang bon tiang thi sao-sao mai prathana," http://www.samunpai.com/sex/show. php?cat=4&id=136 (accessed January 20, 2008).

10. "Phor sami hai kha" [My husband's father gave it to me], http://www.ruengerotic.com/read/70725 (accessed January 20, 2008).

11. "Baem-Bo clear reuang nai 'mung' pert jai kham khoraha sami diao-kan," title of a post by "Baem-Bo," http://hilight.kapook.com/view/6083 (accessed January 20, 2008).

12. "ICTeen Camp: khai yaowachon seu-san reuang phet" [ICTeen Camp: Youth camp for communicating about sexual matters], http://www.plawan.com/content_plawan.php?id=36 (accessed January 20, 2008).

13. Korpkan, "Training Manual" (emphasis in original).

14. "Phu-ying Thai kap reuang thang-phet—khuan pert-phoey di reu mai" [Thai women and reuang phet: Should we divulge them or not?], posted by "Pakang," June 29, 2003, http://board. dserver.org/v/vogel/00000069.html (accessed January 20–25, 2008).

15. C. Panpricha, "Jak panha sukkhaphap jit su panha reuang thang-phet" [From mental health to sexual problems], Cheewajit Magazine, no. 108, April 17, 2004, http://www.bbznet. com/scripts2/view.php?user=healthy&board=4&id=5&c=1&order=numview (accessed January 20–25, 2008).

16. Royal Institute Dictionary of New Words, 59.

17. "Khai 20 khor chuan khorng-jai nai reuang sek khorng phu-ying (reuang sek ngai-ngai thi phu-chai mai ru)," posted by "Pairote39," December 16, 2003, http://www.expert2you.com/view_article.php?art_id=1300 (accessed January 20–25, 2008).

18. "Khru suan yuk mai nun tit krorh ru thao than reuang phet–seu XXX lae AIDS" [Modern Suan Kularp School teachers support wearing a harness of awareness of reuang phet, XXX-rated media and AIDS], Manager Daily, November 30, 2005, http://www.osknetwork.com/modules. php?name=News&file=print&sid=1012 (accessed January 20–25, 2008).

19. Uncyclopedia (Thai edition), s.v. "rok tit sek" [sex addiction], http://th.uncyclopedia. info/wiki/โรคติดเซ็กส์ (accessed January 20–25, 2008).

CHAPTER 2: TO BE CHASTE

1. Kusuma et al., Honor and Shame.

2. See Harrison, "Disruption of Female Desire;" Harrison, "Wild Roses."

3. Sujit Wongthes, "Phut theung 'phet'" [Speaking of "sex"], Miti watthanatham Thai [Dimensions of Thai culture], Manager Online, September 7, 2005, http://chalita.exteen. com/20060421/entry (accessed January 20–25, 2008).

4. Khun Wichitmatra, Thai Idioms.

5. Ibid.

6. Thapani Nakhonthap, Language Informing Us.

7. Khun Wichitmatra, Thai Idioms.

8. Khun Wichitmatra, *Thai Idioms*.

9. *Dictionary of the Royal Institute*, 1999 ed., 401.

10. *Royal Institute Dictionary of New Words*, 68.

11. *Dictionary of the Royal Institute*, 1999 ed., 953.

12. Ibid., 978.

13. *Royal Institute Dictionary of New Words*, 136.

14. *Wikipedia* (Thai edition), s.v. "phasa Thai thin tai" [Southern Thai dialect], http://th.wikipedia.org/wiki/ภาษาไทยถิ่นใต้ (accessed January 20–25, 2008).

15. *Dictionary of the Royal Institute*, 1999 ed., 804.

16. Ibid., 398

17. The Indian tantric ceremony involves a gathering of both female and male worshippers into a temple or a private space. After darkness falls within the space, the male and female parties reach for one other by groping blindly. They are then to have sex with whomever they can grab first, even if the other party is a relative (e.g., father, mother, or sibling) or friend. Ancient scriptures state that it is particularly meritorious if a mother/father/sibling and his or her child/sibling happen to have sex with each other in this ceremony, because it pleases Mother Kali.

18. Kawin, "Dork thorng," February 29, 2008, http://gotoknow,org/blog/kelvin/168214?cla ss=yuimenuitemlabel (accessed September 10, 2007).

19. "Awaiyawa phet ying: Sing saksit andap sorng" [The female sexual organs: second-class sacred objects], posted by "Chai Seri," January 4, 2007, http://www.praphansarn.com/new/forum/forum_posts.asp?PN=34&TID=6127 (accessed September 10, 2007).

20. Some Thai festivals take the form of what anthropologists describe as "rituals of rebellion," when the hierarchies that usually structure polite, respectful, normative behaviour are temporarily overturned in transgressive and often rambunctious play. Festivities for celebrating the Thai new year of Songkran in April and Loi Krathong, the festival of lights held at the end of the wet season on the November full moon, often have this transgressive and playfully rebellious character. Drinking, all-night carousing and partying, as well as casual sex, often take place on the margins of village- or district-level fairs held for these festivals.

21. "Feun kha-niyom 'yaowasatri' 'rak nuan sa-nguan tua' khatha sayop 'mua sek'" [Recovering the values 'young ladies' and *rak nuan sa-nguan tua*: Spelling out the solution for sexual abandon], posted by "Sivakorn," September 27, 2004, http://www.expert2you.com/view_article.php?cat_ sel=129000&art_id=1891 (accessed January 20–25, 2008).

22. Ibid.

23. "Midnight University," adapted from *History of Sexuality* by Michel Foucault, http://www.geocities.com/fineartcmu2001/newpage14 (accessed January 20–25, 2008).

24. Suthida Malikaeo, "Dek tit sek vs. rak nuan sa-nguan tua" [Sex-addicted kids vs. *rak nuan sa-nguan tua*], Kep ma khit, ao ma khian [Thoughts and jottings], *Prachatai*, July 11, 2005, http://www.prachatai.com/05web/th/columnist/viewcontent.php (accessed 20–25 January, 2008).

CHAPTER 3: A WOMANIZER

1. For a translation and commentary of *Khun Chang Khun Phaen*, see Chris Baker and Pasuk Phongpaichit, trans. and eds. *The Tale of Khun Chang Khun Phaen: Siam's Great Folk Epic of Love and War*, 2 vols.

2. *Encarta® World English Dictionary* (North American edition), s.v. "playboy," http://encarta.msn.com/dictionary_/playboy.html (accessed December 11–13, 2007).

3. "Pert horng hi-class" [Opening the hi-class room], *Hi-Class*, issue 69, January 1990, http://www.tuneingarden.com/contentdetail.php?id=CNT_447c2e8cafeb0 (accessed December 11–13, 2007).

4. *Wikipedia* (English edition), s.v. "Giacomo Casanova," http://en.wikipedia.org/wiki/Giacomo_Casanova (accessed December 11–13, 2007).

5. Khun Wichitmatra, *Thai Idioms*, 270.

6. *Dictionary of the Royal Institute*, 1982 ed., 237.

7. There are many versions of *Khun Chang Khun Phaen*, but it is believed that the current *sepha* version was composed in the eras of King Rama II (r. 1809–24) and King Rama III (r. 1824–51). *Chantakorop* is based on rural poetry and was compiled by Sunthorn Phu in the first half of the nineteenth century. *Kaki* was composed by Jao Phraya Phra Khlang also in the nineteenth century.

CHAPTER 4: TO BE A SPINSTER

1. Kanjana Naksakul, *Thai Language Today*, 25.

2. Kanjanakhaphan, *Thai Idioms*, 159.

3. *Dictionary of the Royal Institute*, 1999 ed., 1185.

4. Ibid., 544.

5. *Lan Tham (Larndham) Sewana* [Dharma Forum], 2007, http://larndham.net/index.php?act=Print&client=html&f=4&t=24175 (accessed October 24–29, 2007).

6. "Khwam-mai khorng sao khern" [The meaning of *sao khern*], *Anajak Sao Khern*, March 27, 2006, , http://saokern.is.in.th/?md=content&ma=show&id=1 (accessed October 15, 2007).

7. *Lanna Khadi* [Lanna (Northern Thai) Studies] (Chiang Mai: Mae Jo University, 2007), http://lanna.mju.ac.th/lannafestival_detail.php?recordID=6 (accessed October 24–29, 2007).

8. "Aphichart Jumrutruethirong & Orathai Rucharoenphonphanich" [Sex and the City] (English title spelled phonetically in Thai script), in *Prachakorn lae sangkhom 2550* [Population and Society in 2007], edited by Worachai Thongthai and Suriphorn Phanpheung (Nakhon Pathom, Thailand: Mahidol University, Institute for Population and Social Research, 2007), http://www.ipsr.mahidol.ac.th/content/Home/ConferenceIII/Articles/Article07 (accessed October 24–29, 2007).

9. Post by "Nu Tae," November 11, 2007, http://www.pantip.com (accessed January 16, 2007).

10. Post by "Tua Haeng," November 12, 2007, http://www.pantip.com/cafe/siam (accessed October 24, 2007).

11. Siriphorn Amphaiphong, "Kheun khan phror kan-khoi" [In dry dock because I waited (for you)], song on the music CD album *Klorn rak ruam-samai* [Contemporary Love Ballads], recorded by GMM Grammy, Bangkok, 2001.

12. "Tamnan khan thorng" [The legend of the golden dry dock], November 12, 2005, *Khan-Thong Club*, http://khan-thong-club.exteen.com/ 20051112/ (accessed October 15, 2007).

13. http://www.thaimiss.com/news.php?id=N0114 (accessed October 24–29, 2007). N.B.: Since February 2009, visitors have been warned against entering this site due to a malware concern.

14. S. Kongpeng, "Miss Khan Thorng," July 3, 2006, http://www.fpmconsultant.com/htm/news02.php?id=732 (accessed October 24–29, 2007). N.B.: Sawapha Thephatsadin Na Ayutthaya was the winner of the first Miss Khan Thorng competition in 2003. She may also be the only winner so far, as the competition seems to have been arranged only once. No news was found of any following rounds.

15. Sui Oe, "Thammai torng riak wa khan thorng tha ayu mak mak laeo yang mai taeng-ngan" [Why must old, unmarried women be called *khan thorng*?], http://th.answers.yahoo.com/question/index?qid=20071129071925AOVtR7 (accessed October 15, 2007).

CHAPTER 5: BRIDE PRICE

1. *Dictionary of the Royal Institute*, 1999 ed., 1194.
2. *Royal Institute Dictionary of New Words*, 30.
3. Various explanations have been offered for the meaning of the phrase *sin hua bua nang* in Article 109, section 1 of the *Three Seals Law*. Winai Phongsriphien claims that it comes from calling upper-class men *bua bao* (บัวบ่าว), "lotus youths," and women *bua nang* (บัวนาง), "lotus ladies," which would later have been extended to cover women in general. Khun Wichitmatra, on the other hand, explains that the term referred to the woman's price, with the word *hua* (หัว), "head," referring to the person, and *bua* (บัว), "lotus flower," to the breasts, showing which parts of the woman were seen as valuable. This matches well with the explanation by Phraya Rambanditsithiseranee that "*sin sort* equaled *sin hua bua nang*, or that *sin sort* was a fee for the breasts or milk (*nom*) of the bride." See respectively, Winai Phongsriphien, *Thai Language in the Three Seals Law*; Khun Wichitmatra, *Thai Idioms*; and Phraya Rambanditsithiseranee (1930), cited in Woranat Sribunphong, "Engagement."
4. Cited in Woranat Sribunphong, "Engagement."
5. Ratsada Ekabutr, *Explanations of Family and Engagement Law*.
6. "Khu-rak tom-dee khu nai thi khit ja taeng-ngan kan bang khap" [*Tom-dee* couples: which couples are thinking of getting married?], message no. 27, posted by "Muk," January 7, 2008, http://board.narak.com/topic.php?id=249029 (accessed January 16, 2008).
7. Examples can be found at http://www.weddingsquare.net/#forum/forum_posts. asp? TID=3252.
8. Suriya Rungtawan, "Ten Thousand," song from the motion picture *Love charms of luk thung* [Mon-rak luk-thung], recorded by Saneha Petcharabun, 1970.
9. "Saphai inter" [International daughter-in-law], posted by "Kateul," February 3, 2008, http://www.weddingsquare.com (accessed March 1, 2008).
10. http://www.thaimuslimshop.com/article.php?id=515 (accessed January 20–25, 2008).
11. "Phayaban C5 khriat ni-sin lon tua phuk khor tai kha ror. phor.—thing jot-mai la luk" [Level 5 nurse stressed about debts, hangs herself in the hospital—leaves farewell letter to child], *Matichon Daily*, May 31, 2004.

CHAPTER 6: TO BE SEX-OBSESSED

1. "Luk-chai phor yor. bor. heun–chut sao khom-kheun yap–tor. ror. lai sakat jap dai," *Thai Rath*, October 4, 2007.
2. "Tat-sin 2 khru heun jam khuk 50 pi khom-kheun luk-sit," *Thai Rath*, November 21, 2007.
3. *Dictionary of the Royal Institute*, 1999 ed., 1296.
4. Ibid., 57.
5. "Phu-ying kap phu-chai–khrai heun-kwa kan" [Women and men: who *heun* more?], message no. 1, August 25, 2007, http://www.suanboard.net/view.php?p=view&kid=40989 (accessed October 15, 2007).
6. "Dek-chai keun SK 131," August 25, 2007, http://www.suanboard.net/view.php?p= view&kid=40989 (accessed October 15, 2007).
7. "Theung khiw 'kathoey' heun rum sum!" [Kathoeys turn now to heun and rape!], *Khao Sot*, March 15, 2004, http://www.deedeejang.com/news/news/00166.htm (accessed November 27, 2007).
8. "Rawang phu-ying heun kam kap phu-ying raet–khun mai yak khao klai mak sut?" message no. 1, posted by "Hotaru ka sand," July 11, 2006, http://www.dek-d.com/board/view. php?id=619989 (accessed October 15, 2007).

9. "Rawang phu-ying heun kam kap phu-ying raet–khun mai yak khao klai mak sut?" message no. 7, posted by "Luk kwat si-chomphu11," July 12, 2006, http://www.dek-d.com/board/view.php?id=619989 (accessed October 15, 2007).

CHAPTER 7: TO BE SEX-OBSESSED

1. "The Legendary Midfielder: *Farang–po–thuret* [Westerners–porn–obscene]," May 17, 2006, http://www.bloggang.com/viewdiary.php?id=thenut&month=052006&date=17&group=1&gblog=11 (accessed October 15, 2007).
2. Uncle Fat, "'Ya pow' ja bamrung kamlang torng kin hai thuk thang," [For *ya pow* to increase your stamina, you have to take it correctly], *Manager Daily*, February 24, 2006, http://www2.manager.co.th/Qol/ViewNews.aspx?NewsID=9490000025104 (accessed November 24, 2007).
3. *Dictionary of the Royal Institute*, 1982 ed., 540.
4. *Royal Institute Dictionary of New Words*, 168.
5. Ibid., 58.
6. Matichon, *Non-Royal Institute Dictionary*, 106.
7. Ibid.
8. Thepchu Thapthong, *Life and Background of Thai People*.
9. "Amy ram hai phop or. jor. rap phit—taeng po!" [Amy cries (upon) meeting teacher—admits mistake, she dressed *po*!], *Thai Rath*, February 16, 2007, http://www.thairath.co.th/news.php?section=hotnews&content=37147 (accessed November 24, 2007).
10. See Jackson, "Performative Genders, Perverse Desires."
11. Narupon Duangwises, "Naked Male Models."
12. Nidhi Eoseewong, "The State in Our Beds," 91.

CHAPTER 8: CUNT

1. *Dictionary of the Royal Institute*, 1999 ed., 1294.
2. Raks Thai Foundation, *Reproductive Health*, 67.
3. *Wikipedia* (Thai edition), s.v. "hee" [cunt], http://th.wikipedia.info/wiki/หี (accessed February 1–9, 2008). N.B.: This website has a warning, which states that the article has content unsuitable for children, that young people should use their critical faculties when reading it, and that parents should provide advice.
4. *Uncyclopedia* (Thai edition), s.v. "hee" [cunt], http://th.uncyclopedia.info/wiki/หี (accessed February 1–9, 2008).
5. Ibid.
6. Ibid.
7. This information was obtained through a group discussion with people of diverse sexualities and genders.
8. Ibid.
9. "Sek wittathan–khuat yat jim dap," *Thai Rath*, September 3, 2006, http://www.thairath.co.th/offline.php?section=hotnews&content=18368 (accessed February 1–9, 2008).
10. "Jut sorn-ren reuang leuk . . . leuk tae mai lap!" [The secret spot, a deep issue . . . Deep but not mysterious!], in *Bantheuk Khun Mae* [A mother's notes], no. 163, February 2007, http://www.elib-online.com/doctors50/lady_lady001.html (accessed February 1–9, 2008).
11. ThaiHealth, "Awaiyawa seup-phan satri, kan-du-lae" [Women's reproductive organs care], http://www.thaihealth.net/h/encyclopedia-10073 (accessed February 1–9, 2008).
12. "5 withi pherm khwam-man-jai hai 'norng jim'" [Five ways to increase the confidence

of '*norng jim*'], June 2006, http://www.pooyingnaka.com/story/story.php?Category=sex&No =261 (accessed February 1–9, 2008).

13. Ibid., message no. 38.

14. Khwai Noi, "Ju kap jim" [Willy and fanny], message no. 62, October 27, 2004, http://www.pantown.com/board.php?id=5373&name=board1&topic=245&action=view (accessed September 10, 2007).

15. "Fai boriwen thi lap" [Moles in the area of the *thi lap*], 2007, http://horoscope.sanook.com/mole/ index_secret.php (accessed February 1–9, 2008).

16. "Mor teuan highlight khon thi lap–siang tit cheua" [Doctor warns of doing highlights to pubic hair, risk of infection], http://hilight.kapook.com/view/15823 (accessed February 1–9, 2008).

17. Miro International/Administrator, "Siwaleung" [Shivalinga], 2006, http://www.sriganapati.com/index.php?option=com_content&task=view&id=120&Itemid=46 (accessed February 1–9, 2008).

18. "Khon aphap khu" [A person unlucky with romantic partners], message no. 8, posted by "anothai," October 3, 2005, http://www.thaidoweb.com/freeboard/print.php (accessed September 10, 2007).

19. "Ju jom jap mor-sane hai sao kae pha long na–lup lam khorng sa-nguan," http://hilight.kapook.com/view/6742 (accessed February 1–9, 2008).

20. "Nak-rian por. hok jap pheuan ying kheung pheut tham anajan jap na-ok–khorng sa-nguan" [Sixth-graders hold female friend to ground—commit indecent acts by groping her breasts and *khorng sa-nguan*], http://webboard.mthai.com/5/2006-07-04/248992.html (accessed February 1–9, 2008).

21. "'Ice' sexy tem-thi—Wo! Khor pit khae khornng sa-nguan," November 22, 2007, http://entertain.teenee.com/thaistar/15446.html (accessed February 1–9, 2008).

22. "Jut sorn-ren reuang leuk . . . leuk tae mai lap!" [The secret spot, a deep issue . . . Deep but not mysterious!], in *Bantheuk Khun Mae* [A mother's notes], message no. 163, February 2007, http://www.elib-online.com/doctors50/lady_lady001.html (accessed February 1–9, 2008).

23. Sorajak Siriborirak, "The *khoey* does not itch."

24. "Khan jim" [An itchy *jim*], message no. 1, posted by "anew," October 2, 2004, http://anew.exteen.com/20041002/entry (accessed October 15, 2007).

CHAPTER 9: COCK

1. *Dictionary of the Royal Institute*, 1999 ed., 230.

2. *Ongkhachat* (องคชาต) is a Pali-Sanskrit compound word: *ongkha* (องฺค), n. "organ" + *chat* (ชาต), v. "to be born." Hence, it does not have a vowel symbol on the final consonant, contrary to how many people mistakenly write it: องคชาติ.

3. *Wikipedia* (Thai edition), s.v. "awaiyawa seup-phan chai" [male reproductive organs], http://th.wikipedia.org/wiki (accessed February 15–19, 2008).

4. *Uncyclopedia* (Thai edition), s.v. "khuay" [cock], http://th.uncyclopedia.info/wiki/ควย (accessed February 15–19, 2008).

5. "Rabop seup-phan phet-chai" [The male reproductive system], http://sexclub7.web1000.com/know/sex/know39.html (accessed February 15–19, 2008).

6. *Royal Institute Dictionary of New Words*, 2. In addition to the term *ju*, there is also *norng ju* (น้องจู), which according to a web posting has been defined as "younger brother willy," as in "Umm . . . pants bulging like this. It can be hypothesized to be *norng ju*, no doubt." This expression is often used for a boy's sexual organ. See Niw ma yeuan, "Sangkhang nan . . . samkhan chanai [How

important is jock itch?], message posted September 1, 2006, http://anew.exteen.com (accessed September, 10, 2007).

7. *Royal Institute Dictionary of New Words*, 87.

8. Ibid., 44.

9. Ibid., 86

10. Ibid., 85

11. The Thai original uses roman script for *khuay* here.

12. Bryan Wathabunditkul, "Photjananugay: sap ke gay Thai" [Gay glossary: Cool Thai gay vocabularies], http://www.suphawut.com/gvb/gayly/thai_gay_cultures_gay_vocabs3.htm (accessed October 15, 2007).

13. *Uncyclopedia* (Thai edition), s.v. "khlam" [cock], http://th.uncyclopedia.info/wiki/ขลำ (accessed February 15–19, 2008).

14. Ibid.

15. "Kham thi 1 phasa Isan wan-ni khor-saner kham wa khuay" [Word number 1: Northeastern Thai today is pleased to introduce the word *khuay*], posted by "Teddybear," February 12, 2007, http://www.isan.clubs.chula.ac.th/lang/?transaction=wordbyword.php&Id_lang=532 (accessed February 15–19, 2008).

16. Jintana Malasri, "Khor-patibat thua-pai samrap phu-puai thang rangsiraksa" [General advice for patients undergoing radiation treatment], http://www.geocities.com/suchartW/radiationcare1.htm (accessed February 15–19, 2008).

17. *Wikipedia* (Thai edition), s.v. "dildo," http://th.wikipedia.org/wiki/ดิลโด (accessed February 15–19, 2008).

18. Busakorn, "Khlip nan samkhan chanai" [How important is circumcision?], in *Duang-jai phor mae* [Parents' little darling], no. 125, March 2006, http://www.elib-online.com/doctors49/child_sex001.html (accessed February 15–19, 2008).

19. "Photjananuku" [My dictionary], posted by "nunut," February 7, 2007, http://nunut1984.mobile.spaces.live.com/ent.aspx?b=1&h=cns!D0C9D4D27557AE78!466 (accessed February 15–19, 2008).

20. "Technik kan-tham otthakam samrap phu-chai" [*Otthakam* techniques for men], message no. 1, posted by "Bkknight," November 12, 2003, http://www.bkknight.com/bkkboard/index.php?act=ST&f=8&t=1894 (accessed September 10, 2007).

21. "Ju plorm khorng khrai" [Whose fake dick?], posted by "Mrs. Ruby," www.siamdara.com/column/00000989.html (accessed February 15–19, 2008).

22. For more on *siwaleung*, see "Tamnan siwaleung" [Legend of Shivalinga], messages posted by "Tathen," September 12, 2001, http://board.dserver.org/P/PaKai/00000069.html (accessed September 10, 2007).

23. Phitthaya Bunnag, "Palat khik lae ongkhachat" [*Palat khik* and the phallus], in *Sinlapa Watthanatham*, no. 274, February 1, 2006, http://artgazine.com/shoutouts/viewtopic.php?t=1405 (accessed February 15–19, 2008).

24. "Ju kap jim" [Willy and Fanny], posted by "Khwai noi," message no. 62, October 27, 2004, http://www.pantown.com/board.php?id=5373&name=board1&topic=245&action=view (accessed September 10, 2007).

25. Ibid.

CHAPTER 10: TO BE BUSTY

1. *Royal Institute Dictionary of New Words*, 167.

2. Matichon, *The Non-Royal Institute Dictionary*, 217.

3. "Phiang khae tha cream tua ni Perfect Lift bork la kham wa ok khai dao plian pen kham wa eum dai than-thi," http://classified.sanook.com/item/3104662 (accessed December 1–10, 2007).

4. Helen Burger, "Yoohhoo cover girl," http://www.yoohhoo.com/covergirl2/helen/covergirl.html (accessed September 10, 2007).

5. Post by "botun," February 13, 2007, http://zaaz.name/modules/news/article.php?storyid =95&NewsTab=8 (accessed September 10, 2007). N.B.: The author of the message presents information from a lecture by a female pharmacist working as a development manager for a company offering advice on breasts and breast enlargement services.

6. "Withi serm eum–sai chut suay pai ngan taeng," message no. 1, November 26, 2007, http://www.bloggang.com/mainblog.php?id=everythingon&month=26-11-2007&group=4&gblog=5 (accessed December 10, 2007).

7. "Tata Young sut-eum," message no. 102, posted by "Emma," March 19, 2007, http://www.thainewyork.com/find-473.html (accessed September 10, 2007).

8. "Kratae hong rorn (eum ek sek sutttt)," message no. 1, posted by "Chiaiki," April 7, 2005, http://www.pooyingnaka.com/webboard/show.php?Category=sex&No=4562 (accessed September 10, 2007).

9. "'But' khuang sao yoey khao. . . eum mai phae 'Poey,'" http://www.daradaily.co.th/news_view.aspx?n_id=4422&cat_id=10 (accessed December 1–10, 2007).

10. http://www.blogth.com/blog/Living/Beauty/5805.html (accessed December 1–10, 2007).

11. "Eum," June 8, 2007, http://www.lefthit.com/tag/อึม.html, (accessed December 1–10, 2007).

12. http://www.a-um.com (accessed December 1–10, 2007).

13. Aphilak Kasemphonkun, *Linking the World to Nirvana*, 26.

14. Sor. Phlainoy, "Breasts in Novels."

15. Helen Burger, "Yoohhoo cover girl," http://www.yoohhoo.com/covergirl2/helen/covergirl.html (accessed September 10, 2007).

16. *Royal Institute Dictionary of New Words*, 162–63.

17. "Tata Young sut eum" [Tata Young super-*eum*], message no. 102, posted by "Emma," March 19, 2007, http://www.thainewyork.com/find-473.html (accessed September 10, 2007).

18. Ormsin Saenluan, "Six Tricks to Increase Sexiness," 174.

19. "Yak dai pha rat na-ok a" [I'd like to get a breast-binding strap], posted by "Bugi," June 11, 2007, http://www.lesla.com/board/func_print.php?id=219772&mode_id=3&PHPSESSID=5 8c35565684cda7e94c3add8fa728989 (accessed September 10, 2007) N.B.: As of February 2009, this site was offline.

20. "Show *eum* jaeng kert dai jing reu?" [Can one really announce one's birth (i.e., establishment in the entertainment industry) by showing off *eum*-ness?], posted by "Bugi," http://star.sanook.com/interview/interview_10491.php (accessed December 1–10, 2007).

CHAPTER 11: MALE-TO-FEMALE TRANSGENDERS OR TRANSSEXUALS

1. Jackson, "Male Homosexuality and Transgenderism;" Terdsak Romjumpa, "Discourses on 'Gay' in Thai Society."

2. Ibid.

3. Ibid.

4. Terdsak Romjumpa, "Discourses on 'Gay' in Thai Society."

5. Interview with a female vegetable vendor aged sixty-seven from Thonburi, unmarried, with no formal education.

6. *Dictionary of the Royal Institute Dictionary*, 1999 ed., 93.

7. "Kham thi hen khon riak phuak rao boi-boi" [Words that I see people often call us], posted by "cococurin," May 9, 2006, http://www.thailadyboyz.net/webboard/viewtopic.php?t =1392&postdays=0&postorder=asc&highlight=%BB%C3%D0%E0%B7%D7%CD%A7&sta rt=15 (accessed October 15, 2007).

8. Ibid., post by "mijiru77," May 13, 2006.

9. "Thammai jeung riak kathoey wa tut" [Why are *kathoeys* called *tut*?], message no. 1, posted by "sickboy_1983," July 15, 2007, http://topicstock.pantip.com/library/topicstock/2007/07/ K5579218/K5579218.html (accessed October 15, 2007).

10. Bryan Wathabunditkul, "Photjananugay: sap ke satri lek" [Gay glossary: cool iron ladies vocabularies], http://www.suphawut.com/gvb/gayly/thai_gay_cultures_gay_vocabs2.htm (accessed October 15, 2007).

11. "Hak ja mi kan-banyat sap pheua chai riak transgender yang phuak rao" [If terminology were to be created for describing transgenders like us], posted by "Papillon," December 20, 2006, http://www.thailadyboyz.net/webboard/viewtopic.php?t=4712&highlight=%BB%C3%D0% E0%B7%D7%CD%A7 (accessed October 15, 2007).

12. Jackson, "Male Homosexuality and Transgenderism;" Terdsak Romjumpa, "Discourses on 'Gay' in Thai Society."

13. Vitaya Saeng-aroon and Friends (presenters), *Rai-kan witthayu hotline sai si-rung* ["The Rainbow-Colored Way" radio program], July 28, 2007, Nation Radio Channel FM 97.5. N.B.: The *Rainbow-Colored Way* radio program deals with issues of people of diverse sexualities and genders.

14. Ibid.

CHAPTER 12: WOMEN WHO LOVE WOMEN

1. Jackson, *Dear Uncle Go*.

CHAPTER 13: MEN WHO LOVE MEN

1. Terdsak, "Discourses on 'Gay' in Thai Society."

2. Jackson, "Tolerant but Unaccepting."

3. Vitaya Saeng-aroon, "Fang laeo yoey" [When I hear it—ew!], Lerk aep sia thi [High time to come out of the closet], *Manager Online*, May 26, 2004. N.B.: This website was not operative as of February 2009.

4. "Tham kan jang pen ruk reu rap" [Always asking if we're *ruk* or *rap*], posted by "skinny-head," March 25, 2007, http://www.thaimalemassage.com (accessed October 15, 2007).

5. Ibid., post by "smart_guy 69."

6. Ibid., post by "skinnyhead."

CHAPTER 14: PROSTITUTES

1. "Kan kha praweni," http://th.wikipedia.org/wiki/การค้าประเวณี (accessed October 15, 2007).

2. Dararat Mattariganond, "Prostitution and the Thai Government's Policies."

3. Ibid.

4. "Kha-niyom mi kik tham khon tit AIDS phung–mae ban siang sung sut" [The practice of having a *kik* makes the number of people infected with AIDS skyrocket—housewives at greatest risk], http://www.policehospital.go.th/main/view.php?group=2&id=183&PHPSESSID=4fab 58a32f5b649 (accessed October 15, 2007).

CHAPTER 15: TO HAVE SEX

1. *Dictionary of the Royal Institute,* 1999 ed., 920.
2. *Wikipedia* (Thai edition), s.v. "eup" [to shag], http://th.wikipedia.org/wiki/อึ๊บ (accessed October 15, 2007).
3. *Dictionary of the Royal Institute,* 1999 ed., 700.
4. *Lum dam* [The black hole], Burapha TV, Bangkok Channel 9, January 17, 2007.
5. "Sor. Nor. Chor. phan kot-mai phua ham khom-kheun mia" [NLA (National Legislative Assembly) passes law banning husbands from raping their wives], http://hilight.kapook.com/view/12380 (accessed October 15, 2007).

CHAPTER 16: TO ACHIEVE ORGASM

1. Bryan Wathabunditkul, "Photjananugay: sap ke satri lek" [Gay glossary: cool iron ladies vocabularies), http://www.suphawut.com/gvb/gayly/thai_gay_cultures_gay_vocabs2.htm (accessed October 15, 2007).
2. Dr. Sukamol Wiphawiphakul, http://www.smustsay.com/sexmustsay_2005 (accessed October 15, 2007).
3. Ibid.
4. "Mi sek yang-ngai hai set (theung jut sut-yort)" [How can I have sex to achieve orgasm (reach the highest point)?] message no. 1, posted by "d . . . da," May 19, 2006, http://www.pooyingnaka.com/webboard/show.php?Category=sex&No=6830 (accessed October 15, 2007).

CHAPTER 17: TO MASTURBATE

1. *Nation Sut Sapda,* vol. 8, no. 370, July 29–August 4, 1999.
2. *Klai mor,* vol. 25, issue 8, August, 2001.
3. "Khu-meu phu-sorn rai wicha 'Phet-seuksa'" [Teacher's manual for the subject of "sex education"], 2004, http://www.teenpath.net/teenpath/manual/manual03-03-01.doc (accessed October 15, 2007).
4. *Krungthep Wan-athit,* vol. 16, no. 5995, November 21, 2003.
5. Phansak Sukrarerk, "Sat khorng kan-mi khwam-suk duay tua-eng" [The science of having happiness with yourself], *Nation Sut Sapda,* vol. 8, no. 370, July 29–August 4, 1999.
6. Ibid.
7. "Khu-meu phu-sorn rai wicha 'Phet-seuksa'" [Teacher's manual for the subject of "sex education"], 2004, http://www.teenpath.net/teenpath/manual/manual03-03-01.doc (accessed October 15, 2007).
8. "Chuay tua-eng . . . khwam-jampen thi seu-sat kap thuk khon" [*Chuay tua-eng . . .* loyal necessity for all people], http://www.clinicrak.com (accessed October 15, 2007).
9. Personal communication with Waen, a twenty-seven-year-old corporate employee, April 6, 2008.
10. *Wikipedia* (Thai edition), s.v. "kan-samret khwam-khrai" [achieving sexual gratification], http://th.wikipedia.org/การสำเร็จความใคร่ (accessed October 15, 2007).
11. "Chuay tua-eng . . . khwam-jampen thi seu-sat kap thuk khon" [*Chuay tua-eng . . .* loyal necessity for all people], http://www.clinicrak.com (accessed October 15, 2007).
12. "Khu-meu phu-sorn rai wicha 'Phet-seuksa'" [Teacher's manual for the subject of "sex education"], 2004, http://www.teenpath.net/teenpath/manual/manual03-03-01.doc (accessed October 15, 2007).
13. http://www.smustsay.com/sexmustsay_2005/sexbox/inner.php?level=2&id=46 (accessed October 15, 2007).

14. Dr. Phansak Sukrarerk, "Sat khorng kan-mi khwam-suk duay tua-eng" [The science of having happiness with yourself], *Nation Sut Sapda*, vol. 8, no. 423, July 10–16, 2000.

CHAPTER 18: TO HAVE ORAL SEX

1. *Nation Sut Sapda*, vol. 9, no. 67, May 14–20, 2001.
2. *Krungthep Thurakij*, February 15, 2000.
3. Jackson, "Male Homosexuality and Transgenderism."
4. Bryan Wathabunditkul, "Photjananugay: sap ke gay Thai" [Gay glossary: cool Thai gay vocabularies], http://www.suphawut.com/gvb/gayly/thai_gay_cultures_gay_vocabs3.htm (accessed October 15, 2007).
5. Prawit Phisanbutr, *Warasan Clinic*, September, 1999, 48.
6. *Nation Sut Sapda*, vol. 9, no. 67, May 14–20, 2001.
7. Ibid.
8. http://www.kachon.com/board/index.php? (accessed October 15, 2007).
9. *Nation Sut Sapda*, vol. 9, no. 67, May 14–20, 2001.
10. Cited in *Nation Sut Sapda*, vol. 9, no. 67, May 14–20, 2001.
11. Prawit Phisanbutr, *Warasan Clinic*, September 1999, 48.

CHAPTER 19: TO SODOMIZE

1. R. Saisuk, "Thi-ma khorng kham wa 'thua dam'" [Origins of the word *thua dam*], July 5, 2006, http://knowledge.eduzones.com/knowledge-2-14-44206.html (accessed October 15, 2007).
2. "Jap khru makan tui dek ni kop dan Thai 5 pi. Khom Chat Leuk," October 27, 2006, cited in "Wa duay khwam-pen-ma khorng kham wa tui" [On the origins of the word *tui*], http://parininospace.spaces.live.com/blog/cns!B7D8F81BFBBBF70D!114.entry (accessed October 15, 2007).
3. "Sor. sor. tui long mai kiao dek-chai yeua kam—Pramot taeng ngiap setthini Phuket," *Matichon Daily*, February 14, 1998, cited in "Wa duay khwam-pen-ma khorng kham wa *tui*" [On the origins of the word *tui*], http://parininospace.spaces.live.com/blog/cns!B7D8F81BFBBBF 70D!114.entry (accessed October 15, 2007).
4. "Khru tui thua dam phlik lin patiset thuk khor-ha," *Siam Rath*, March 20, 1998, cited in "Wa duay khwam-pen-ma khorng kham wa tui" [On the origins of the word *tui*], http://parininospace.spaces.live.com/blog/cns!B7D8F81BFBBBF70D!114.entry (accessed October 15, 2007).
5. Cited in Jackson, *Dear Uncle Go*, 151; Sarakadee Editorial Board, "From *Thua Dam* to *Tui*," 855.
6. "Num khaen–mao lap thuk gay lak 'tui' rua ying mai yang tai kha talat," *Khao Sot*, September 11, 2004.
7. "Pi ni pi seua bai–jak tui C8 ton tamrap theung khru tui nor. ror. yok chan–phor tui luk dor. chor. 4 khuap," *Khao Sot*, March 1, 1998.
8. "Khru rap tui dek khoey ok hak kliat phu-ying," *Matichon Daily*, March 19, 1998.
9. Bryan Wathabunditkul, "Photjananugay: sap ke gay Thai" [Gay glossary: cool Thai gay vocabularies], http://www.suphawut.com/gvb/gayly/thai_gay_cultures_gay_vocabs3.htm (accessed October 15, 2007).
10. "Wa duay khwam-pen-ma khorng kham wa tui" [On the origins of the word *tui*], http://parininospace.spaces.live.com/blog/cns!B7D8F81BFBBBF70D!114.entry (accessed October 15, 2007).

CHAPTER 20: PARTNER SWAPPING

1. "Khwam-mai khorng kham wa 'swinging'" [The meaning of the word *swinging*], http://dict.truehits.net/?search=swinging (accessed October 15, 2007).

2. http://th.kapook.com (accessed October 15, 2007).

3. Phaet Sandot, *The Partner-Swapping Game*, 35.

4. Ibid., 36.

5. *Khom Chat Leuk*, August 22, 2006, 2.

6. Ibid.

7. "Eung! Web 'swinging' jai member 5 phan mao ror. ror. mua party" [Amazing! A *swinging* website sells membership for five thousand [baht]—hotel rented for wild [sex] parties], http://hilight.kapook.com/view/14720 (accessed October 15, 2007).

8. Ibid.

9. http://www.swingstory.com (accessed October 15, 2007). N.B.: By February 2009, this website had been forced offline by a court order.

10. http://th.kapook.com (accessed October 15, 2007).

11. Wiriya Sathirakul, "Thalai rang swinging–salap khu! Jap 'Kangfu' Thai *Playboy*," [Nest of swingers busted! "Kangfu" of Thai *Playboy* arrested!], *Khom Chat Leuk*, November 5, 2004, http://www.komchadluek.net/column/scup/2004/11/05.php (accessed October 15, 2007).

12. Ibid.

13. http://www.thaimental.com/modules.php?name=news&file=article&sid=281 (accessed October 15, 2007).

14. Message posted by "Ying," August 7, 2007, http://board.narak.com/topic.php?No=148396 (accessed October 15, 2007).

15. Dr. Phansak Sukrarerk, "Suk kap sek: Swinging kheu aria" [Suk (author's pen name) and sex: What is *swinging*?], *Khom Chat Leuk*, April 1, 2005.

CHAPTER 21: A CASUAL PARTNER

1. Department of Curriculum and Instruction Development, *The Creation of a Slang Dictionary*.

2. *Royal Institute Dictionary of New Words*, 11.

3. The original Thai version did not state the names of the authors of the study, but they are given in the media report detailed in note 4 below. A book with the same title as this study was also published. See P. B. N'JOIN, "*Kik*": *More Than a Friend But Not a "Faen."*

4. "Wijai nisit Chula. phop 10 niyam 'kik' ti-phae rak wai rian" [Chulalongkorn University students' research finds ten definitions for *kik*—interpreted as meaning teen love], *Matichon Daily*, January 12, 2004. The article summarizes the research project as follows: "Chula students search for a definition of *kik* among students, report it to be very popular now, quite like a *chu* (ชู้), 'secret lover,' because one can have an unlimited number even if one has a *faen* (แฟน), 'partner;' [it is considered] more than a *pheuan* (เพื่อน), 'friend,' but not a *faen*; said to add flavor (*rotchat*) to life, to be vitamins for the heart."

5. *Wikipedia* (Thai edition), s.v. "kik" [casual partner], http://th.wikipedia.org/wiki/กิ๊ก (accessed January 20–25, 2008).

6. "Wijai nisit Chula. phop 10 niyam 'kik' ti-phae rak wai rian" [Chulalongkorn University students' research finds ten definitions for *kik*—interpreted as meaning teen love], *Matichon Daily*, January 12, 2004.

7. Department of Curriculum and Instruction Development, *Creation of a Slang Dictionary*.

8. *Royal Institute Dictionary of New Words*, 104.

9. "Kae roi 'sap jo' phasa Thai 2002" [Tracing the origins of Thai youth slang, 2002], *Matichon Daily*, April 17, 2002, http://www.matichonbook.com/newsdetail.php?gd=44614 (accessed January 20–25, 2008).

10. See, e.g., *Royal Institute Dictionary of New Words*; Matichon, *Matichon Dictionary of the Thai Language*.

11. *Wikipedia* (Thai edition), s.v. "kik" [casual partner], http://th.wikipedia.org/wiki/กิ๊ก (accessed January 20–25, 2008).

12. See *Dictionary of the Royal Institute*, 1999 ed., 1178, 817, 256, and 815, respectively. Translator's note: It is noteworthy that the only definition given here for *faen* is the distinctive Thai sense of a romantic partner. This dictionary does not refer to the original meaning of "fan" in English as "admirer" or "enthusiast" as in music fan, movie fan, boxing fan, etc.

13. "Kham wa 'kik' kheu rai" [What does the word *kik* mean?], message no. 1, posted by "waeo," September 27, 2004, http://www.365jukebox.com/script/ms/music/m14210 (accessed September 10, 2007).

14. Ibid., message no. 3.

15. Ibid., message no. 7.

16. Ibid., message no. 10.

17. "Wijai nisit Chula. phop 10 niyam 'kik' ti-phae rak wai rian," [Chulalongkorn University students' research finds ten definitions for *kik*—interpreted as meaning teen love], *Matichon Daily*, January 12, 2004.

18. "Kham wa 'kik' kheu rai" [What does the word *kik* mean?], message no. 2, posted by "Mati," September 28, 2004, http://www.365jukebox.com/script/ms/music/m14210.html (accessed September 10, 2007).

19. "Kham wa kik khun khao-jai yang-rai" [How do you understand the word *kik*?], message no. 1, posted by "Phu-yai," June 23, 2006, http://web board.mthai.com/7/2006-06-23/246481. html (accessed October 10, 2007).

GLOSSARY AND INDEX OF THAI TERMS

The Thai terms in this glossary and index are alphabetized according to roman transcription, followed by the Thai script in parentheses, the register of usage (e.g, colloquial, formal, etc.), the literal translation (set off in quotation marks), and finally, common meanings if different from the literal translation. For example, *chak wao* (ชักว่าว), colloquial, "to fly a kite," a euphemism for male masturbation. Following each term are the page number(s) where the term is cited in the text.

A

aep jit (แอบจิต), slang, a "sneaky mind/heart," a closeted gay man, a "closet queen," 129

aep yu (แอบอยู่), slang, "to live secretly," to be closeted, used for gay men, 129

ai (ไอ้), a masculine term that often has a derogatory sense when prefixed to other terms and expressions; compare with *ee*, 81, 90, 93–95, 114

ai jiao plorm (ไอ้เจี๊ยวปลอม), slang, a "fake willy," a dildo, 94

ai jorn (ไอ้จ้อน), slang, the "little guy," the penis, 94

ai khuay (ไอ้ควย), colloquial/crude, "cock," "dick," 93. See also *khuay*

ai na hee (ไอ้หน้าหี), slang/crude, "cuntface," a strong term of abuse for a man, 81

ai nan (khorng phu-chai) (ไอ้นั่น[ของผู้ชาย]), slang, "that thing" (of a man), the penis, 95

ai ngo (ไอ้โง่), slang/crude, "you fuckwit!," strong expression of abuse, 93

ai sat (ไอ้สัตว์), slang/crude, "you animal!," strong expression of abuse, 93

ai wen (ไอ้เวร), slang/crude, "damn you!," strong expression of abuse, 93

Anjaree Group (อัญจารี), Thailand's oldest NGO promoting the rights of women who love women. More recently, the group's advocacy work has extended to promoting the rights of all people of diverse genders and sexualities in Thailand. The name is coined from two Pali terms, *anya* (อัญญ, "to be other" or "to differ") and *jari* (จารี, "to travel" or "move"), and means "to follow a different path," 12, 118–19, 125

antha (อัณทะ), formal, "testicles," 89–91, 95

ao kan (เอากัน), colloquial, "to take it," to have sex, 3, 19, 145, 148–49, 169 *attakamakiriya* (อัตกามกิริยา), formal, "masturbation," 156

at thua dam (อัดถั่วดำ), slang/derogatory, "to stuff black beans," a crude expression for anal sex between men, 127–28, 168–69

awaiyawa khorng phu-ying (อวัยวะของผู้หญิง), "women's [sexual] organs," 83

awaiyawa phet (อวัยวะเพศ), "sexual orgasm," 83–84, 86, 89–90, 92, 94

awaiyawa phet phai-nork (อวัยวะเพศภายนอก), "external sexual organs," 83

awaiyawa seup-phan (อวัยวะสืบพันธุ์), formal, "reproductive organs," 28, 79, 83, 86, 89, 94

awaiyawa seup-phan chai (อวัยวะสืบพันธุ์ชาย), formal, "male reproductive organs," 89, 94

awaiyawa seup-phan satri (อวัยวะสืบพันธุ์สตรี), formal, "female reproductive organs," 83

B

bak ham noi (บักหำน้อย), Northeastern Thai, "little balls," an affectionate expression for a young boy, 93

bak khuay (บักควย), Northeastern Thai/crude, "you dickhead!," an expression of abuse, 93

bambat khwam-khrai duay ton-eng (บำบัดความใคร่ด้วยตนเอง), formal/academic, "to treat/relieve/desire by oneself," to masturbate, 156

bao khern (บ่าวเคิ้น), Northern Thai, an "old bachelor," 51

bao thao (บ่าวเถ้า), Northern Thai, an "old bachelor," 51

berk phrommajan (เบิกพรหมจรรย์), obsolete, "to open the hymen," an ancient Cambodian ritual marking a girl's transition to sexual maturity, 35

beum (บึ่ม), slang, an onomatopoeic word used in expressions emphasizing the size of a man's penis, 92

both (Thai pronunciation: *bot*) (โบ๊ธ), colloquial, from the English word "both," a sexually versatile gay man who engages in both receptive and insertive anal sex, 21, 129–31

buap (บ๊วบ), gay slang for performing oral sex, 163

bua pheuan (บัวเผื่อน), gay slang for performing oral sex, 163

bua riang (บัวเรียง), gay slang for performing oral sex, 163

bukkhon biang-ben thang-phet (บุคคลเบี่ยงเบนทางเพศ), medical/pathologizing, "a sexually deviant individual," 116

burut-phet (บุรุษเพศ), formal, the "male sex" of humans, 27

C

Casanova (Thai pronunciation: *khasanowa*) (คาสซาโนว่า), borrowed from the name of the historical figure, a ladies' man, a lady-killer, 44–48

chai chatri (ชายชาตรี), colloquial, "he-man," 39

chai lin (ใช้ลิ้น), colloquial, "to use the tongue," to perform cunnilingus, 163

chai pak (ใช้ปาก), colloquial, "to use the mouth," to perform oral sex, 162–63, 165, 167

chai rak chai (ชายรักชาย), "men who love men," sometimes used to translate "men who have

dek khai tut (เด็กขายตูด), colloquial/crude, a "kid who sells his ass," a male sex worker who performs receptive anal sex with a male client, 138

dek la taem (เด็กล่าแต้ม), slang, a "point-chasing kid," a young woman who seeks to "score" as many sexual conquests with men as she can in order to impress her friends, 146

dek mok (เด็กโม๊ก), colloquial, a "kid who performs oral sex," a male sex worker who fellates a male client, 138. See also *mok*

dek sideline (Thai pronunciation: *dek sai-lai*) (เด็กไซด์ไลน์), colloquial, a "sideline kid," a young man or woman who engages in sex work part-time, as a "sideline," 137

dek tit sek (เด็กติดเซ็กส์), colloquial, a "sex-addicted kid," denotes teenage sex seen as a social problem, an expression used in campaigns against sex among youth, 33

dek wang (เด็กวัง), slang, a "palace kid," a sex worker working the streets around the Grand Palace area of Bangkok, 136

do (โต๊ะ), slang, "to fuck," a term used by *gays*, 171

doi trong (โดยตรง), slang, "directly," a term used by *kathoey* sex workers to denote male clients with a sexual preference for transgender and transsexual partners, 138

dork thorng (ดอกทอง), slang/derogatory, "golden flower," a slut, used for women regarded as sexually active; also used ironically within *gay* and *kathoey* cultures to denote a sexually active person seen as indiscriminate in their choice of sexual partners, 38–39, 46, 135, 140

dorng thork (ดองถอก), colloquial, a penis that has the foreskin pulled back, 38

dut (ดูด), slang, "to suck up into the mouth," to perform oral sex, 163

dut hoi (ดูดหอย), slang, "to suck the shellfish," to perform cunnilingus, 163. See also *hoi*

E

ee (อี), a feminine term that often has a derogatory sense when prefixed to other terms and expressions; used to denote women as well as *kathoeys* and effeminate gay men; compare with *ai*, 82, 93, 135–36

ee aep (อีแอบ), slang/derogatory, a "damned closet case," used within gay communities to denote a closeted gay man, a "closet queen," 127, 129. See also *aep jit*

ee hee wai (อีหีไว), slang/crude/derogatory, "you fast/instant cunt!," an expression of abuse for women considered to have many sexual partners, 82

ee hee yort rian (อีหียอดเหรียญ), slang/crude/derogatory, "you coin-op cunt!," an expression of abuse for a female sex worker, 82

ee khuay (อีควย), Northeastern Thai/slang/crude/derogatory, "you dickhead!," 93

ee nu (อีหนู), slang/often derogatory, a young female prostitute; *nu* ("little mouse") is an expression for a young girl, 136

ee pi (อีปิ้), slang, "shrimp paste," the female genitals, 87

ee tua (อีตัว), slang/derogatory, a female prostitute, 135, 140

ek (เอ็กซ์), (Thai pronunciation of the letter "X": *ek*), colloquial, "pornography," abbreviated from the English word "X-rated," 70, 99 *erotic* (อีโรติค), (Thai pronunciation: *irotik*), colloquial, from the English, used to denote erotic art and aesthetic eroticism, contrasted with pornographic materials, which are labeled as *po*, 70–71

eum (อึ่ม), colloquial, (of women) "to be busty," "to have large breasts," 98–105

eup (อึ๊บ), *eup kan* (อึ๊บกัน), slang, "to have sex," 19, 145–46

F

faen (แฟน), colloquial, a romantic and sexual partner, may denote a boyfriend, girlfriend, husband, wife, partner, etc.; from the English word "fan," as in a "sports fan," 61, 85, 180–83, 185

fai rap (ฝ่ายรับ), colloquial, the "receptive partner," used in both *gay* and *tom-dee* communities to denote the sexually receptive partner in either male-male or female-female sex, 115, 122, 130

fai ruk (ฝ่ายรุก), colloquial, the "active partner," used in both *gay* and *tom-dee* communities to denote the sexually active partner in either male-male or female-female sex, 122, 130, 152

fan (ฟัน), slang/crude, "to cut/slash," to have sex, 146

fan dap (ฟันดาบ), colloquial, "to fence (with swords)," used in *gay* communities to denote male-male sex, 169. See also *dap*

fan laeo thing (ฟันแล้วทิ้ง), slang/crude, "to fuck and run," 146

fu (ฟู), slang, in *gay* communities, denotes a large, erect penis, 92

G

gay (เกย์), from the English, a gay man, xiv–xv, 6, 8, 11–12, 91, 110–11, 115, 126–32, 170

gay king (เกย์คิง), from the English, the sexually active partner in a *gay* relationship; now somewhat dated and replaced by *fai ruk*, 8, 18, 21, 130

gay queen (เกย์ควีน), from the English, the sexually receptive partner in a *gay* relationship; now somewhat dated and replaced by *fai rap*, 8, 21, 130

gay quing (เกย์ควิง), abbreviated from the English term "gay *queen-king*," a sexually versatile gay man; now somewhat dated and replaced by *both*, 130

H

haen (แฮ่น), Northern Thai/slang, to behave in a flirtatious and dissolute way, 38

haet (แฮด), Northeastern Thai/slang, to behave in a flirtatious and dissolute way, 38. See also *raet*

hai tha (ให้ท่า), colloquial, "to flirt," 65

ham (ห่ำ), colloquial, the "balls," "scrotum," 92–93, 95

hee (ที), colloquial/crude in many contexts, "cunt," the female sexual organs, 19–20, 79–82, 86, 88, 96 *hee haek* (หีแหก), colloquial/crude/derogatory, "torn cunt," an expression of abuse, 81

hee khiao (หีเคียว), Northeastern Thai/colloquial/crude/derogatory, "sickle cunt," to behave in a flirtatious and dissolute way, 38, 81

hee lae (หีแหล่), colloquial/crude, denotes a woman with black or darkly colored sex organs, implying a woman who has had so much sex that her sexual organs have turned dark or black, 81

her hee (เห่อหี), colloquial/crude, "cunt crazy," an expression of abuse, 81

heun (หืน), *heun kam* (หืนกาม), colloquial, "to be sex mad," "sex-obsessed," 18, 64–68

Hinayana (หินยาน), the "lesser path," another term for Theravada Buddhism, 80

hoi (หอย), colloquial, "shellfish," a euphemism for the female sexual organs, 86, 88

hok-sip hok ror. dor. (66 ร.ด.), slang, an indirect euphemism for *raet*, 37

hor mok (ห่อหมก), slang, the name of a Thai dish of steamed fish in curry paste, in *gay* communities refers to a man's large penis visible through his trousers, 91

hua pok (หัวโปก), colloquial, "shaven head," a *kathoey* who wears her hair short, 113, 115

J

jai thao hee mot (ใจเท่าหีมด), colloquial/derogatory, "[to have] a heart the size of an ant's cunt," 81

jampi (จำปี), a flower whose shape is regarded as being reminiscent of the male genitals; a euphemism for the penis, 94

jao chu (เจ้าชู้), a "womanizer," 43, 46–49

jao chu kai jae (เจ้าชู้ไก่แจ้), colloquial, a man who shows off his *jao chu*, i.e., womanizing behavior, compared to a bantam rooster, *kai jae*, strutting about to show his interest in hens, 46

jao chu pratu din (เจ้าชู้ประตูดิน), obsolete, *pratu din* is the name of an inner gate on the Tha Tien side of the Grand Palace in Bangkok. In the past, men were not allowed to enter the royal palace through this gate and, therefore, those with a taste for palace ladies, called *jao chu pratu din*, had to congregate outside this gate to court such women, 46

jao chu yak (เจ้าชู้ยักษ์), colloquial, a "giant *jao chu*" means a man who courts women inconsiderately or outright violently, like giants (*yak*) in Thai classical drama, 46

jao jampi (เจ้าจำปี), colloquial, "lord *jampi*," a euphemism for the penis, 94–95. See also *jampi*

jao lok (เจ้าโลก), colloquial, "lord of the world," a euphemism for the penis, 91, 94, 97

ji (จี๋), variant of *jim*, 87

jiao (เจี๊ยว), colloquial, "willy" (UK), "dick" (US), the penis, 90, 94

jim (จิ๋ม), colloquial, "fanny" (UK), "pussy" (US), the female genitals, 5, 19, 82, 84–88, 94, 97

jo (โจ๊ะ), slang, "to fuck," a term used by *gays*, 171

jop sin (จบสิ้น), colloquial, "to bring to an end," to achieve orgasm, 150 *jor khai daeng* (เจาะไข่แดง), slang, "to pierce the egg yolk," for a man to sexually penetrate a woman, 146

ju (จู๋), colloquial, "willy" (UK), "dick" (US), the penis, the male genitals, 5, 85, 88, 90, 94, 97

jut sorn-ren (จุดซ่อนเร้น), colloquial, "hidden spot," the female genitals, 82–83, 86–87

K

K. (เค), slang, the English letter "K," in *gay* communities, a euphemism for the penis, from the first letter of the romanized spelling *khuay* (cock), 92

kai (ไก่), slang, "hen," "chick," a prostitute, 136

kai sanam luang (ไก่สนามหลวง), slang, a "Sanam Luang chick," a female sex worker who works from the street in the Sanam Luang area of Bangkok, 137

Kaki (กากี), a figure from Thai classical literature, used disparagingly to refer to women regarded as sexually dissolute, 17, 39, 47

kam (กาม), formal/academic, "sexual desire," 28, 64

kamarok (กามโรค), formal/academic, "sexual diseases," 139

kamarom (กามารมณ์), formal/academic, "sexual desire," 28, 64

kan-chai pak (การใช้ปาก), colloquial, "using the mouth," to perform oral sex, 162–63, 165, 167

kan-laek khu (การแลกคู่), "switching/exchanging sexual partners," 175

kan-laek-plian khu-norn (การแลกเปลี่ยนคู่นอน), "switching/exchanging sexual partners," 175

kan-luluang (การลุล่วง), "achievement," to achieve orgasm, 150

kan mi phet-samphan korn wai an khuan (การมีเพศสัมพันธ์ก่อนวัยอันควร), formal/academic, "having sex before an appropriate age," underage sex, 40

kan-ruam-phet (การร่วมเพศ), formal, "to engage in sexual intercourse," 28

kan-salap khu-norn (การสลับคู่นอน), "switching/exchanging sexual partners," 175

kan-samret (การสำเร็จ), "successful completion," a euphemism for orgasm, 150

kan-tham rak duay pak (การทำรักด้วยปาก), formal, "making love with the mouth," to perform oral sex, 162

kapi (กะปิ), slang, "shrimp paste," the female genitals, 87

karaoke (คาราโอเกะ), (Thai pronunciation: *kharaoke*), slang, a euphemism for performing fellatio, comparing the microphone held close to the mouth while performing karaoke to the penis, 163

kathoey (กะเทย), derogatory in some contexts, a trans-woman; male-to-female transgender or transsexual, 6–7, 9, 11, 16, 19, 21, 37, 51, 66–68, 81-82, 109–17, 120–21, 123, 125–28, 132–33

kathoey thae (กะเทยแท้), formal/academic, a "genuine *kathoey*," an intersex person, 110

kep sabu (เก็บสบู่), slang, "to pick up the soap," derived from Western motion pictures that portray male prisoners dropping a bar of soap in the shower and bending over to pick it up, which Thai audiences mistakenly interpret as showing a readiness to have sex, 171

khaek (แขก), "guest," "customer," used by sex workers to denote a male client

khaek chorp hai cho (แขกชอบให้โชว์), slang, an "exhibitionist customer," used among female and transgendered sex workers, 138

khaek doi (แขกโดย), slang, a "direct customer," used by *kathoey* sex workers to denote a client who has a sexual preference for transgender and/or transsexual partners; abbreviated from *doi trong*, 138

khaek kin ngu (แขกกินงู), slang, a "client who eats the snake," used by *kathoey* sex workers to denote clients who like to perform oral sex on pre-operative transsexual partners, 138

khaek ngi-ngao (แขกงี่เง่า), slang, a "stupid customer," used among transgendered sex workers, 138

khaek norng ni (แขกน้องนี), slang, used by *kathoey* sex workers to refer to the customers of female sex workers, 138. See also *chani*

khaek rok-jit (แขกโรคจิต), slang, a "psycho customer," used by *kathoey* sex workers to refer to clients regarded as having bizarre sexual tastes, 138

khaem lek (แคมเล็ก), "labia minora," at the mouth of the vagina, 79, 84

khaem yai (แคมใหญ่), "labia majora," larger than the labia minora and outside of them, 80, 84

khai (ไข่), colloquial, "eggs," refers to the testicles, or "balls," 91, 93, 95

khai dao (ไข่ดาว), colloquial, "'fried egg breasts," denotes flat breasts, 98

khai issara (ขายอิสระ), "freelance" sex workers, 137

kha mia (ค้าเมีย), colloquial, "wife trading," to engage in wife swapping, 173

kham-phet (ข้ามเพศ), "transgender and/or transsexual," 10, 13

kha nam nom (ค่าน้ำนม), "breast milk fee," a synonym for *sin sort*, 57

khanika (คณิกา), obsolete, a "prostitute," 134

khao khang lang (เข้าข้างหลัง), colloquial, "to enter from behind," to perform anal sex or perform sex from behind, 169

khao pratu lang (เข้าประตูหลัง), slang, "to enter by the back door," to perform anal sex, 169

khat jaruat (ขัดจรวด), slang, "to polish the rocket" (of men), to masturbate, 157

khat kha dorng (คาดค่าดอง), Northeastern Thai, "setting the price of becoming related," a synonym for *sin sort*, 59

kheun khan (ขึ้นคาน), colloquial, "to go into dry-dock," used in reference to a woman who remains unmarried, equivalent to the English word "spinster," 18, 22, 50, 52–56

kheun khru (ขึ้นครู), colloquial, "to approach the teacher" of heterosexual men, to have their first sexual experience with a woman; denotes the sexual initiation of young heterosexual men, often with a female sex worker, 22, 141

kraju (กระจู๋), slang, "willy," "dick," a variant of *ju*, 90

krapok (กระโปก), slang, "scrotum," 94

krari (กระหรี่), colloquial, a female or *kathoey* sex worker, 38, 135, 140

krasan (กระสัน), "to lust," "to crave," 65

krathiam (กระเทียม), slang, "garlic," a slang term for *kathoey*, 113

kratuk moi (กระตุกหมอย), slang, "to jerk the pubes" (of males), to masturbate, 157

kratung-krating (กระตุ้งกระติ้ง), "to be effeminate," "to be sissy," 132

kunlagay (กุลเกย์), a "socially respectable gay man," derived from *kunlasatri*, 130

kunlasatri (กุลสตรี), a "socially respectable woman," who follows traditional norms of sexual propriety, 7, 22, 34–35, 46, 52, 80–81, 84, 130, 146, 152–53, 159

L

ladyboy (เลดี้บอย), colloquial, from English, a synonym for *kathoey* often used by Thais when speaking with foreigners, 113–14

lakkaphet (ลักเพศ), formal, "to steal [another's] sex," a transvestite, 127–28

lang (asuji) (หลั่ง[อสุจิ]), "to ejaculate (sperm)," 150

lang na kai (ล้างหน้าไก่), slang, "to wash the chicken's face" (of men), to masturbate in the morning when waking up with an erection, 157

len hu len ta (เล่นหูเล่นตา), colloquial, "to play with the ears and eyes," to flirt, 65

len pheuan (เล่นเพื่อน), obsolete, "to play with a friend," used in the past for female-female sexual relations, 119–20, 147

len sawat (เล่นสวาท), obsolete, "to play at love," used in the past for male-male sex, especially denoting anal sex between men, 127

len siao (เล่นเสียว), colloquial, "to play thrills," female masturbation, 157

les (เลส), slang, from "*les*bian," a woman in a romantic and sexual relationship with another woman; in some instances denotes a woman who does not necessarily engage in the typical gender roles as either a masculine tom or feminine *dee*; in other instances *les* may be understood as a feminine lesbian and conflated with *dee*, 8, 122–23

lesbian (เลสเบี้ยน), from English, a term that Thai women who love women (*ying rak ying*) tend to avoid using because of its associations in Thailand with pornography for heterosexual men, 20, 119, 121–22

les king (เลสคิง), slang, from "*les*bian" and "gay *king*," a lesbian who is the sexually active partner, 8, 123

les queen (เลสควีน), slang, from "*les*bian" and "gay *queen*," a lesbian who is the sexually receptive partner, 8, 123

leung (ลึงค์), from the Sanskrit word *linga*, the phallus, especially in the religious context of *Siwa-leung* (Shivalinga), the symbolic phallus of the Hindu god Shiva, 27, 95, 97

lia (เลีย), slang, "to lick," to perform cunnilingus, 163

lia hoi (เลียหอย), slang, "to lick the shellfish," to perform cunnilingus, 163. See also *hoi ling* (ลิงค์), variant of *leung*, 27

long lin (ลงลิ้น), slang, "to dip the tongue," to perform cunnilingus, 163

M

mae mai (แม่ม่าย), a "widow," 50, 60

mai (ไม้), slang, "wood," "stick," "rod," a euphemism for the penis, 91–92

mai pa diao-kan (ไม้ป่าเดียวกัน), colloquial, "trees in/from the same forest," an old expression for male-male sex, 127

masturbation (มาสเตอร์เบชั่น), from English, the term has been borrowed into Thai and is used with the same meaning, 156, 158

mia (เมีย), "wife," 112, 183–84

mia noi (เมียน้อย), a "minor wife," an unofficial second wife, 45, 174, 182

mi chu (มีชู้), "to have a secret lover" (of a married woman), for a woman to have sex with a man who is not her husband, 184. See also *chu*; *pen chu*

mi sek kan (มีเซ็กส์กัน), colloquial, "to have sex," 169

mok (โม๊ค), slang, abbreviated from the English word "smoke," to perform fellatio, 138, 169

Mora (โมรา), a figure in Thai classical literature who had several husbands, used disparagingly to refer to women regarded as sexually dissolute, 47

mot luk (มดลูก), the "uterus," 79

MSM (เอ็มเอสเอ็ม), from the English acronym "MSM," with the same meaning, "men who have sex with men," 126–27, 130, 132, 155

N

nai (นาย), "Mr.," the Thai title used before men's names, 56

nakhorn sopheni (นครโสเภณี), obsolete, a "city beauty," a term used in the past for a female sex worker, 134

nak-rak (นักรัก), colloquial, a "good lover," usually used by men who pride themselves on their skill as lovers, 152

nak-seuksa sao sideline (นักศึกษาสาวไซด์ไลน์), slang, a "sideline student," a female high school or university student who engages in part-time sex work, as a "sideline," 137

nam taek (น้ำแตก), slang, "water breaks out" (of men), to ejaculate, 150

nang (นาง) "Mrs.," the Thai title used before the names of married women, 56

nang bang ngao (นางบังเงา), colloquial, "lady hiding in the shadows," a female sex worker working from the streets at night, 135

nang klang meuang (นางกลางเมือง), colloquial, "downtown lady," a euphemism for a female sex worker, 153

nang lom (นางโลม), colloquial, "comfort lady," a female sex worker, 135

nang-ngam rong-raem (นางงามโรงแรม), colloquial, a "hotel beauty," a female sex worker working from a hotel, 136 *nang-ngam tu krajok* (นางงามตู้กระจก), colloquial, a "glass-case beauty," a female sex worker working from a massage parlor where the workers wait for clients in a room fronted with a glass wall, 136

nang sao (นางสาว), "Miss," the Thai title used before the names of unmarried women, 56, 114

nang thang-thorasap (นางทางโทรศัพท์), colloquial, a "telephone lady," a call girl or female sex worker who is contacted by clients by phone, 136

nang thian (นั่งเทียน), slang, "to sit on the candle," refers to anal sex involving sitting on a man's erect penis, 171

na ok na jai (หน้าอกหน้าใจ), the (female) "breasts," 102

ngian (เงี่ยน), slang, "to be randy" (UK), "to be horny" (US), 65

nok-khao (นกเขา), slang, a "dove," the penis, 90

nok-khao mai khan (นกเขาไม่ขัน), slang, the "dove doesn't coo," a euphemism for male impotence, 90

nok-krajork kin nam (นกกระจอกกินน้ำ), slang, the "sparrow drinks water," premature ejaculation, 90

nok-krajork mai than kin nam (นกกระจอกไม่ทันกินน้ำ), slang, the "sparrow isn't fast enough to drink water," premature ejaculation, 90

nom yai (นมใหญ่), "big breasts," 99

norn kan (นอนกัน), "to sleep together," to have sex, 146

norng chai (น้องชาย), colloquial, "little brother," a euphemism for the male genitals, 90, 95

norng jim (น้องจิ๋ม), colloquial, "little sister *jim*," variant of *jim*, 84, 87

norng nang thang ha (น้องนางทั้ง 5), slang, "all the five young ladies," a euphemism for male masturbation, with "five young ladies" referring to all five fingers of a hand used to stroke the penis, 156

norng sao (น้องสาว), colloquial, "little sister," a euphemism for the female genitals, 87

norng toey (น้องเตย), slang, "younger sibling *toey*," a young *kathoey*, 113

nude (นู้ด), borrowed from the English word with the same meaning, usually used in the context of art or photographic images, 70–71

nu jim (หนูจิ๋ม), colloquial, "little *jim*," variant of *jim*, 87

num sideline (หนุ่มไซด์ไลน์), colloquial, "sideline boy," a young man who engages in part-time sex work, as a "sideline," 137

O

oi (อ่อย), "to be lustful," "to seduce," 65

om (อม), colloquial, "to suck and hold in the mouth," a euphemism for performing fellatio, 163

om kluay (อมกล้วย), slang, "to suck on the banana," to perform fellatio, 163

ongkhachat (องคชาต), formal/academic, "penis," "phallus," 89–90, 94, 96

P

phet-saphap (เพศสภาพ), academic, "gender" (lit. *"phet* status"), 11

phetsarot (เพศรส), formal, "sexual tastes," 28

phet-sat (เพศศาสตร์), academic, "sexology," 28

phet-seuksa (เพศศึกษา), academic, "sex education," 28, 121

phet thi-sam (เพศที่สาม), the "third sex," a *kathoey*, 116

phet-withi (เพศวิถี), academic, "sexuality" (lit. *"phet* orientation"), 11, 13, 125

phi khanun (ผีขนุน), slang, a "jackfruit ghost," a female or *kathoey* sex worker who works from the streets around the Khlong Lot area of Bangkok, where there are many jackfruit *(khanun)* trees, 136

phi makham (ผีมะขาม), slang, a "tamarind ghost," a female sex worker who works from the streets in the Sanam Luang area of Bangkok, where there are many tamarind *(makham)* trees, 137

phit phet (ผิดเพศ), academic/medical, "wrong-sexed," "wrong-gendered," variously used to refer to transgenderism, transsexualism, and homosexuality, which are regarded as pathologies within Thai professional medical and psychology circles, 120

phraya the khrua (พระยาเทครัว), slang/obsolete, a womanizing man, 44

phrommajan (พรหมจรรย์), formal, "celibacy," 22, 35

phrommajari (พรหมจารี), formal, (of women), "virginity," "chastity," 35

phuang sawan (พวงสวรรค์), colloquial, the "heavenly bunch," a euphemism for the male sex organs; can be compared with the English term "family jewels," 91, 95

phu-chai (ผู้ชาย), a "man," usually denotes a heterosexual man and is used in contrast to *gay*, xiv–xv, 4, 6, 16, 46, 109, 115

phu-chai dork mai (ผู้ชายดอกไม้), colloquial, a "flower man," a *kathoey* or gay man, 128

phu-chai khai nam (ผู้ชายขายน้ำ), colloquial, a "man who sells water," a male sex worker, 138

phu-chai mi hee (ผู้ชายมีหี), slang/derogatory, a "cunt of a man," 81

phu-chai na ya (ผู้ชายนะยะ), colloquial, a "na ya man," a kathoey or effeminate gay man, 127, 129

phu-chai pai leuang (ผู้ชายป้ายเหลือง), colloquial, a "yellow sign man," a male sex worker, 138

phu-chai si-muang (ผู้ชายสีม่วง), colloquial, a "lavender man," an effeminate gay man, 128

phu-ying (ผู้หญิง), woman, usually denotes a heterosexual woman, contrasted with a *tom*, xii, xiv, 4, 6, 16, 109, 122, 139

phu-ying ha kin (ผู้หญิงหากิน), colloquial, a "working woman," a euphemism for a female sex worker, 135

phu-ying kham-phet (ผู้หญิงข้ามเพศ), a "cross-gender woman" or "transgender woman," a recent alternative expression for *kathoey*, 114

phu-ying praphet sorng (ผู้หญิงประเภทสอง), colloquial, a "second type of woman," a more polite term than *kathoey* for male-to-female transgenders and transsexuals, xv

phu-ying yam cha (ผู้หญิงหยำฉ่า), colloquial, a "tearoom woman," a female sex worker who works from a Chinese tearoom, 136 *pi* (ปิ๊), slang, "shrimp paste," the female genitals, 87

pi kan (ปิ๊กัน), colloquial, "to have sex," 19, 145

pla khem (ปลาเค็ม), slang, "salted fish," the female genitals, 87

playboy (เพลย์บอย), colloquial, from the English and used as a synonym for *jao chu*, 44–45, 48

po (โป๊), colloquial, "to be pornographic," 17, 22, 69–75

Pratheuang (ประเทือง), slang/derogatory, a recent alternative for *kathoey*, from the title of a 1999 pop song, 113–14

praweni (ประเวณี), formal, "to have sexual relations," 147

pu mia (ปู่เมีย), Northern Thai/obsolete, a regional expression for *kathoey*, 112

pum krasan (ปุ่มกระสัน), colloquial, the "lust button," the clitoris, 86

R

raet (แรด), slang, a "rhinoceros," to behave in a dissolute and flirtatious way, 17, 37–38, 46, 67

raet lop nai (แรดหลบใน), slang, "to *raet* covertly," 37

raet ngiap (แรดเงียบ), slang, "to *raet* quietly," 37

rak diao jai diao (รักเดียวใจเดียว), "to love only one person," 46, 48

rak nuan sa-nguan tua (รักนวลสงวนตัว), idiom, "to love and reserve one's body," to be and remain chaste, 17, 22, 33–37, 39–41, 46, 48, 71, 101–2, 146, 152, 177, 179

rak phet diao-kan (รักเพศเดียวกัน), "to love the same sex," 13

rak-ruam-phet (รักร่วมเพศ), biomedical/often pathologizing term to refer to "homosexuality," now resisted by Thai LGBT groups and replaced by *rak phet diao-kan* ("same-sex love"), 13, 66, 128

ran (ร่าน), (sexually) "to want," "to lust after," 17, 37, 46, 65, 81

rap (รับ), (sexually) "to be receptive/passive," 130–31

reuang bon tieng (เรื่องบนเตียง), colloquial, "matters in bed," sexual relations, 28

reuang nai mung (เรื่องในมุ้ง), colloquial, "matters within the mosquito net," sexual relations, 28–29

reuang phet (เรื่องเพศ), "sexual matters," 1, 3, 27, 29–33

reuang sek (เรื่องเซ็กส์), "sexual matters," 29–33

reuang tai sadeu (เรื่องใต้สะดือ), colloquial, "matters below the belly button," sexual matters, 28–29

reuang thang-phet (เรื่องทางเพศ), "sexual matters," 29

reuang yang wa (เรื่องอย่างว่า), colloquial, "that kind of thing/those kind of things," a euphemism for sexual matters, 28–29

rok phu-chai (โรคผู้ชาย), "men's diseases," an expression coined by some feminists for sexually transmitted diseases (STD) in order to resist the implication of the common expression *rok phu-ying* that women alone are the source of STDs, 140 *rok phu-ying* (โรคผู้หญิง), colloquial, "women's diseases," a common expression for sexually transmitted diseases, 139

rok tit-tor thang-phet-samphan (โรคติดต่อทางเพศสัมพันธ์), formal, "sexually transmitted diseases," 139

rorng (ร่อง), slang, "furrow," "groove," a euphemism for the female sexual organs, 86

rorng sawat (ร่องสวาท), slang, "love furrow," a euphemism for the female sexual organs, 86

ruk (รุก), (in sexual relations), slang, "to be insertive/active," 115, 130–31

rup po (รูปโป๊), a "pornographic image," 69

S

salai norn (สไลด์หนอน), slang, "to slide the worm," a euphemism for male masturbation, 156

salit (สะหลิด), Northern Thai/slang, "to behave in a flirtatious and dissolute way," 38

salua jit (สลัวจิต), slang, a "dimly illuminated mind," a closeted gay man who is unsuccessful in attempting to hide his homosexuality, 129

samana-phet (สมณเพศ), formal, refers to the religious status of an ordained Buddhist monk, 27

sami (สามี), formal, "husband," 182–83

samret khwam-khrai duay ton-eng (สำเร็จความใคร่ด้วยตนเอง), formal, "to satisfy desire by oneself," to masturbate, 156–57, 159

samsorn (สำส่อน), "to be promiscuous," 139, 186

sangwat (สังวาส), formal/obsolete, "sexual intercourse," 147

sao kae (สาวแก่), an "old maid," "spinster," 50–51

sao kamphaeng din (สาวกำแพงดิน), colloquial, a "Kamphaeng Din girl," a female sex worker working from the Kamphaeng Din red light area of Chiang Mai city in northern Thailand, 136

sao khern (สาวเคิ้น), Northern Thai, an "unmarried woman," 51

sao oke (สาวโอเกะ), slang, a "karaoke girl," a female sex worker who works from a karaoke bar, 136

sao praphet sorng (สาวประเภทสอง), colloquial, a "second type of young woman," a more polite term than *kathoey* for younger male-to-female transgenders and transsexuals, 13, 20–21, 81, 100, 102, 112–16, 125–26, 133, 136

sao rong nam-cha (สาวโรงน้ำชา), colloquial, a "tearoom girl," a young female sex worker who works from a Chinese tearoom, 136

sao siap (สาวเสียบ), slang, a "penetrating girl," a pre-operative male-to-female transgender or transsexual who plays the sexually active role with a male partner, 21, 113, 115

sao thao (สาวเฒ่า/สาวเถ้า), an "old maid," "spinster," 51

sao theua (สาวเทื้อ), colloquial, an "old maid," "spinster," 50–51

sao theum theuk (สาวทึมทึก), colloquial, an "old maid," "spinster," 50 *satri bamrer* (สตรีบำเรอ), colloquial, "entertainment lady," a euphemism for a female sex worker, 135

satri-phet (สตรีเพศ) formal, (of humans) the "female sex," 27

sawang jit (สว่างจิต), slang, a "brightly illuminated mind," an out gay man, 129

sek (เซ็กส์), borrowed from the English word "sex," in the sense of "to have sex," 31, 147

sek eua-athorn (เซ็กส์เอื้ออาทร), slang, "charity sex," group sex and/or partner swapping, 175

sek mu (เซ็กซ์หมู่), colloquial, "group sex," 175

sep sangwat (เสพสังวาส), formal/obsolete, "to have sexual intercourse," 147

sep som (เสพสม), colloquial, "to have sex," 147

set (เสร็จ), colloquial, "to finish," to achieve orgasm, 18, 116, 150–55

seua phu-ying (เสือผู้หญิง), colloquial, a "lady tiger," a lady killer, synonym for *Casanova*, 44–45

seu lamok anajan (สื่อลามกอนาจาร), formal, "obscene publications/media," 72

seu yua-yu thang-phet (สื่อยั่วยุทางเพศ), "sexually provocative material," 70

sexy (เซ็กซี่), borrowed from English with the same meaning, 70–71, 74, 99

sia (khwam) sao (เสีย[ความ]สาว), "to lose one's maidenhood," to lose one's virginity, 146

siap (เสียบ), slang, "to penetrate," used by *gays* and *kathoeys* to denote anal sex, 171

sia tua (เสียตัว), colloquial, "to lose oneself" or "to be damaged," to lose one's virginity, 19, 36, 58, 146

sideline (ไซด์ไลน์), (Thai pronunciation: *sailai*), slang, borrowed from the English, to engage in part-time sex work, as a "sideline," 137

sik (ซิก), slang, "to penetrate," used among *gays*, 171

sin sort (สินสอด), "bride price," 22, 57–63

sip-et ror. dor. (11 ร.ด.), slang, a synonym for *raet*, 37

sopheni (โสเภณี), a "prostitute," 7, 18, 20, 22, 134–35, 140

sort(sai) (สอด[ใส่]), "to penetrate" sexually, 59

suan nan (ส่วนนั้น), colloquial, "that part," a euphemism for the genitals, 87

suang ok (ทรวงอก), formal, the "breasts," 101

swinger (สวิงเกอร์), slang, from English, a person who engages in partner swapping, 173, 175, 179

swinging (สวิงกิ้ง), slang, from English, to engage in partner swapping, xiv, 18, 22–23, 72, 173–79

T

taek (แตก) slang, "water/semen breaks out," (of men) to ejaculate, 150, 152

taeng-tua po (แต่งตัวโป๊), "to dress provocatively/revealingly," 69

taeo (แต๋ว), slang, a *kathoey* or effeminate gay man, 113 *taet* (แตด), colloquial, the "clitoris," 86

tam taeng (ตำแตง), slang, "to pound the cucumber," male masturbation, 157

tao nom (เต้านม), the "breasts," 101–2

TG (ทีจี), from the English acronym for transgender, recently adopted in some *kathoey* circles to denote a male-to-female transgender or transsexual person, 113–14

thaeng ai tim (แท่งไอติม), slang, an "ice cream stick," the penis, 95

thaeng hareuhan (แท่งหฤหรรษ์), slang, "joystick," the penis, 95

tham (ถ้ำ), slang, a "cave," the vagina, 86

theung (ถึง), colloquial, "to reach," to achieve orgasm, 152

theung jut sut-yort (ถึงจุดสุดยอด), colloquial, "to reach the highest point," to achieve orgasm, 150, 152

theung sawan (ถึงสวรรค์), colloquial, "to reach heaven," to achieve orgasm, 150

thi lap (ที่ลับ), colloquial, a "secret place," the genitals, 20, 86–87

thi na pheun noi (ที่นาผืนน้อย), slang, a "small rice paddy," the female genitals, 87

thua dam (ถั่วดำ), slang, "black beans," anal sex between men, 138, 168–69

ti ching (ตีฉิ่ง), slang, "to beat cymbals," sex between women, 122, 147

tok bet (ตกเบ็ด), slang, "setting the fishhook," female masturbation, 157

tom (ทอม), colloquial, from "*tom*boy," a masculine woman whose romantic and sexual partner is a *dee*; a masculine lesbian, 6, 8, 18, 60, 103, 110–11, 119, 121–23, 127

tom one-way (ทอมวันเวย์), colloquial, a *tom* who is strictly the sexually active with a *dee* partner, 122

tom two-way (ทอมทูเวย์), colloquial, a *tom* who will permit a *dee* partner to be the sexually active party, 122

torm luk mak (ต่อมลูกหมาก), the "prostate gland," 89

torm sang nam liang asuji (ต่อมสร้างน้ำเลี้ยงอสุจิ), "seminal vesicles," tubular glands that secrete a significant portion of the fluid that eventually becomes the semen, 89

transgender (ทรานส์เจนเดอร์), from the English, with the same meaning, 114

trong nan (khorng phu-ying) (ตรงนั้น [ของผู้หญิง]), colloquial, "right down there" (for a woman), a euphemism for the female genitals, 86

tua diao an diao (khorng phu-chai) (ตัวเดียวอันเดียว[ของผู้ชาย]), slang, "(a man's) one and only," the penis, 95

tui (ตุ๋ย), slang/usually derogatory, anal sex between men, 127–28, 168–71

tuk tuk (ตุ๊กตุ๊ก), slang, a "(jerky) three-wheel motor taxi," denotes the jerky hand movement of male masturbation, "to jerk off," 157

tum (ตุ้ม), slang, an onomatopoeic word used to refer to the large size of a man's penis, 92

tut (ตุ๊ด), slang/derogatory, "poofter" [UK], "faggot" [US], 12–13, 66, 113, 127

U

umong sawat (อุโมงค์สวาท), slang, "love tunnel," the vagina, 86

W

Wanthorng (วันทอง), a female figure from Thai classical literature, used disparagingly to refer to women regarded as sexually dissolute, 17, 47, 49

Y

(ya) ching suk korn ham ([อย่า] ชิงสุกก่อนห่าม), idiom, "don't rush ripeness before half-ripeness," don't engage in premarital sex, save oneself for marriage, 36

ye (เย), slang/crude, "to fuck," adapted from *yet*, used by *gays*, 147, 171

ye kan (เยกัน), slang, "to have sex," used by *gays, 169*

yet (เย็ด), slang/crude, "to fuck," 147, 171

yeua phrommajan (เยื่อพรหมจรรย์) or *yeua phrommajari* (เยื่อพรหมจารี), formal, the "hymen," 80

ying khom khiao (หญิงโคมเขียว), colloquial, "woman of the green lantern," a female sex worker in early modern Bangkok, when brothels were required to be identified by a green lantern hung at the front of the establishment, 135

ying nakhorn sopheni (หญิงนครโสเภณี), obsolete, a "woman of the city," a female prostitute, 134

ying ngam haeng nakhorn (หญิงงามแห่งนคร), obsolete, a "beautiful woman of the city," a female prostitute, 134–35

ying ngam meuang (หญิงงามเมือง), obsolete, a "beautiful woman of the city," a female prostitute, 134–35

ying P. (หญิงพี), colloquial, a "P. woman," a euphemism for a female prostitute, using the first letter of the English word "prostitute," 140

ying rak ying (หญิงรักหญิง), "women who love women," 4, 8, 13, 20, 118–23, 125–27, 129

yok kha (ยกขา), slang, "to lift the legs," to prepare for analingus, or anal sex, where the receptive party lifts up the legs, to be penetrated by anal sex, used by *gays*, 171

yok sot (ยกซด), slang, "to raise [a glass/noodle bowl] to drink," to lift up the buttocks to prepare for analingus or to be penetrated in anal sex, used by *gays*, 163

yoni (โยนี), formal, the "female genitals," 86

BIBLIOGRAPHY

Aphilak Kasemphonkun. *Linking the World to Nirvana* [Phuk nipphan loki]. Bangkok: Matichon, 2007. In Thai.

Baker, Chris and Pasuk Phongpaichit, trans. and eds. *The Tale of Khun Chang Khun Phaen: Siam's Great Folk Epic of Love and War.* 2 vols. Chiang Mai: Silkworm Books, 2010.

Bourdieu, Pierre. *Distinction: A Social Critique of the Judgement of Taste.* Translated by Richard Nice. London: Routledge and Kegan Paul, 1984.

Dararat Mattariganond. "Prostitution and the Thai Government's Policies 1868–1960" [Sopheni kap nayobai khorng rathaban Thai Phor. Sor. 2411–2503]. Unpublished master's thesis, Chulalongkorn University, Bangkok, 1983. In Thai.

Department of Curriculum and Instruction Development, Ministry of Education. *The Creation of a "Slang Dictionary": A Manual for the Study of Slang* [Naeo-thang kan-jat-tham "photjananukrom kham khanorng" khu-meu kan-seuksa kham khanorng]. Bangkok: Ongkan Kha Khurusapha, 2000. In Thai.

Fairclough, Norman. *Discourse and Social Change.* Cambridge, UK: Polity Press, 1992.

Harrison, Rachel V. "The Disruption of Female Desire and the Thai Literary Tradition of Eroticism, Religion and Aesthetics." *Tenggara* 41 (2000): 88–125.

———. "Wild Roses and Urban Boring Bees: (Western) Feminist Readings of a Thai Feminine Text?" *Tenggara* 47/48 (2004): 93–115.

Harrison, Rachel V. and Peter A. Jackson, eds. *The Ambiguous Allure of the West: Traces of the Colonial in Thailand.* Hong Kong: Hong Kong University Press, 2010.

Jackson, Peter A. "An American Death in Bangkok: The Murder of Darrell Berrigan and the Hybrid Origins of Gay Identity in 1960s Thailand." *GLQ: A Journal of Lesbian and Gay Studies* 5, no. 3 (1999): 361–411.

———. *Dear Uncle Go: Male Homosexuality in Thailand.* Bangkok: Bua Luang, 1995.

———. "Male Homosexuality and Transgenderism in the Thai Buddhist Tradition." In *Queer Dharma: Voices of Gay Buddhists,* edited by Winston Leyland, 55–89. San Francisco: Gay Sunshine Press, 1998.

———. "Performative Genders, Perverse Desires: A Bio-History of Thailand's Same-Sex and Transgender Cultures." *Intersections: Gender, History and Culture in the Asian Context* 9 (2003), http://intersections.anu.edu.au/issue9/jackson.html.

———. "Thai Research on Male Homosexuality and Transgenderism and the Cultural Limits of Foucaultian Analysis." *Journal of the History of Sexuality* 8, no. 1 (1997): 52–85.

———. "Tolerant but Unaccepting: The Myth of a Thai 'Gay' Paradise." In *Gender and Sexualities in Modern Thailand*, edited by Peter A. Jackson and Nerida Cook, 226–42. Chiang Mai, Thailand: Silkworm Books, 1999.

Kanjanakhaphan. *Thai Idioms* [Samnuan Thai]. Bangkok: Bamrungsat Publishers, 1979. In Thai.

Kanjana Naksakul. *The Thai Language Today* [Phasa Thai wan-ni]. Bangkok: Pheuan Di Press, 2001. In Thai.

Khun Wichitmatra [Sa-nga Kanjanakhaphan]. *Thai Idioms* [Samnuan Thai]. Bangkok: School of Language and Culture, Technology Promotion Association (Thailand-Japan), 2000. In Thai.

Korpkan Mahatthano. "Training Manual for Friends' Corner Youth Camp Leaders" [Khu-meu kan-op-rom khai kaen-nam mum pheuan jai wai-run]. Nonthaburi, Thailand: Reproductive Health Division, Department of Health, Ministry of Public Health, 2004. In Thai.

Kusuma Raksamani, Saowanit Chulawong, and Saiwarun Noinimit. *Honor and Shame in Thai Literature* [Saksi lae khwam-ap-ai nai wannakam Thai]. Bangkok: Maekhampang Press, 2007. In Thai.

Martin, Fran, Peter A. Jackson, Mark McLelland, and Audrey Yue, eds. *AsiaPacifiQueer: Rethinking Gender and Sexuality in the Asia-Pacific.* Urbana and Chicago: University of Illinois Press, 2008.

Matichon. *Matichon Dictionary of the Thai Language* [Photjananukrom chabap Matichon]. Bangkok: Silpa Watthanatham, 2004. In Thai.

———. *The Non-Royal Institute Dictionary* [Photjananukrom nork Ratchabandit]. Bangkok: Matichon, 2000. In Thai.

Narupon Duangwises. "Naked Male Models: Porn Books and Sexual Desire in the Lives of Thai *Gays*." [Pleuay nai baep: nang-seu po lae kamarom nai chiwit gay Thai]. *Ratthasatsan* 25, no. 2 (2005): 173. In Thai.

Nidhi Eoseewong. "The State in Our Beds" [Rat bon tiang norn]. *Matichon Sut Sapda*, vol. 27, no. 1406, July 27–August 2, 2007, 91–92. In Thai.

Ojanen, Timo. "Sexual/Gender Minorities in Thailand: Identities, Challenges, and Voluntary-Sector Counselling." *Sexuality Research and Social Policy* 6, no. 2 (2009): 4–34.

Ormsin Saenluan. "Six Tricks to Increase Sexiness" [6 khlet lap pherm khwam-sexy]. *Thai Cosmopolitan*, no. 127, October 2007, 174. In Thai.

P. B. N'JOIN. *"Kik": More Than a Friend But Not a "Faen"* [Kik mak-kwa pheuan tae mai chai faen]. Bangkok: Rawang Banthat, 2004. In Thai.

Phaet Sandot [pseud.]. *The Partner-Swapping Game* [Game laek khu]. Bangkok: Anongsin Printers, 1982. In Thai.

Raks Thai Foundation. *Reproductive Health and Choices for the HIV Positive: Guidelines for Counseling* [Anamai jarernphan lae thang-leuak samrap phu tit cheua HIV: Naeo-thang kan-hai borikan preuksa]. Bangkok: Lake and Fountain Printing, 2007. In Thai.

Ratsada Ekabutr. *Explanations of Family and Engagement Law* [Kham-athibai kotmai khrorp-khrua–kan-man]. Bangkok: Winyanchon Press, 2005. In Thai.

Royal Institute of Thailand. *Dictionary of the Royal Institute, 1982 edition* [Photjananukrom chabap Ratchabandittayasathan phor. sor. 2525]. Bangkok: Samnak-phim Aksorn Jarernthat, 1998. In Thai.

———. *Dictionary of the Royal Institute, 1999 edition* [Photjananukrom chabap Ratchabandittayasathan phor. sor. 2542]. Bangkok: Nanmee Books Publications, 2003. In Thai.

————. *Principles of Transcribing Thai Phonetically in Roman Script* [Lak-ken kan-thort aksorn Thai pen aksorn roman baep thai siang], 1999, http://www.royin.go.th/upload/246/FileUpload/416_2157.pdf. In Thai.

————. *Royal Institute Dictionary of New Words* [Photjananukrom kham mai lem 1 chabap Ratchabandittayasathan], Vol. 1. Bangkok: Mac, 2007. In Thai.

Sarakadee Editorial Board. "From *Thua Dam* to *Tui*" [Jak thua dam theung tui]. In *108 Envelopes of Questions* [108 sorng kham-tham lem], Vol. 8. Bangkok: Sarakadee Press, 2000. In Thai.

Siriphorn Amphaiphong. "In Dry Dock Because I Waited (for You)" [Kheun khan phror kankhoi]. Song on the album *Contemporary Love Ballads* [Klorn rak ruam-samai]. Bangkok: GMM Grammy, 2001. In Thai.

Sor. Phlainoy [pseud.]. "Breasts in Novels" [Nom nai niyai]. In *Men and Women* [Phu-ying, phu-chai]. Bangkok: Pimkham, 2001. In Thai.

Sorajak Siriborirak. "The *Khoey* Does Not Itch" [Reuang khoey mai khan]. *Phraeo*, vol. 16, no. 381, July 10, 1995. In Thai.

Suriya Rungtawan. "Ten Thousand" [Sip meun]. Song from the motion picture *Love Charms of luk thung* [Mon-rak luk-thung]. Recorded by Saneha Petcharabun. Bangkok: Rungsuriya Phaphayon, 1970. In Thai.

Terdsak Romjumpa. "Discourses on 'Gay' in Thai Society, 1965–1999" [Wathakam kiao-kap "gay" nai sangkhom Thai phor. sor. 2508–2542]. Unpublished master's thesis, Chulalongkorn University, Bangkok, 2002. In Thai.

————. "From '*Kathoey*' to '*Gay*': The History of Male Homosexuals in Thai Society" [Jak "kathoey" theung "gay" prawattisat chai rak-ruam-phet nai sangkhom Thai]. *Warasan Aksorasat* 31, no. 1 (2003): 303–35. In Thai.

Thapani Nakhonthap. *Language Informing Us—From "Kor. Kai" to "Hor. Nok Huk": 200 Idioms* [Phasa–pha-san aksorn kor. kai—hor. nok huk 200 samnuan]. Bangkok: Bannakit, 1980. In Thai.

Thepchu Thapthong. *The Life and Background of Thai People in the Past* [Chiwit lae khwam-lang khorng khon Thai samai-korn]. Bangkok: Prasertwathin Publications, n.d. In Thai.

Van Esterik, Penny. *Materializing Thailand*. Oxford: Berg, 2000.

————. "Repositioning Gender, Sexuality, and Power in Thai Studies." In *Genders and Sexualities in Modern Thailand*, edited by Peter A. Jackson and Nerida M. Cook, 275–89. Chiang Mai, Thailand: Silkworm Books, 1999.

Wierzbicka, Anna. *Understanding Cultures Through Their Key Words: English, Russian, Polish, German, and Japanese*. Oxford: Oxford University Press, 1997.

Williams, Raymond. *Keywords: A Vocabulary of Culture and Society*. New York: Oxford University Press, 1976.

Winai Phongsriphien, ed. *The Thai Language in the Three Seals Law* [Phasa Thai nai kotmai tra sam duang]. Bangkok: Samlada, 2007. In Thai.

Woranat Sribunphong. "Engagement: Analysis of its Special Characteristics and Legal Consequences" [Kan-man: Wikhror laksana phiset lae phon thang kotmai]. Unpublished master's thesis, Thammasat University, Bangkok, 1991. In Thai.

CONTRIBUTORS

PIMPAWUN BOONMONGKON is Associate Professor and the Director of the Center for Health Policy Studies at Mahidol University, Salaya Campus. She also teaches at Thammasat University. Her research interests include sexuality, gender, and sexual and reproductive health. In addition, Dr. Boonmongkon is an executive committee member of the Southeast Asian Consortium on Gender, Sexuality, and Health. Together with academics from six other institutions in Southeast Asia, she co-founded the consortium in 2003 to develop a body of knowledge on gender, sexuality, and health in the region. She serves as the main presenter for the consortium's short leadership courses on gender, sexuality, and health, including international courses in English and bilingual programs conducted in Thai and Lao. Dr. Boonmongkon received her Ph.D. in Medical Anthropology from the University of California, San Francisco-Berkeley.

PETER A. JACKSON is Professor of Thai Cultural Studies in the Australian National University's College of Asia and the Pacific. He has written extensively on modern Thai cultural history with special interests in religion and sexuality. He is Editor-in-Chief of the *Asian Studies Review* and founder of the Thai Rainbow Archives Project, which is collecting and digitizing Thai gay, lesbian, and transgender magazines and community organization newsletters (see http://thairainbowarchive.anu.edu.au/index.html). He received his Ph.D. from ANU in 1987. His most recent book is *Queer Bangkok: 21st Century Markets, Media and Rights* (Hong Kong University Press and Silkworm Books, 2011).

MONRUEDEE LAPHIMON is an activist, an independent researcher, and a training course facilitator on issues of HIV/AIDS, gender, and sexuality. She currently works on HIV/AIDS, gender, sexuality, and women's health issues. Previously, she worked as a project coordinator for the Southeast Asian Consortium on Gender, Sexuality, and Health. Most recently, she collaborated in research with the Center for Health Policy Studies. She was also one of the founders of the Thai Women and HIV/AIDS Task Force, an independent working group born of the collaborative efforts of women with an interest in HIV/AIDS and women's health and rights. She holds a master's degree from Chiang Mai University.

NIWAT KONGPHIAN is the editor of the *Music Journal* published by Mahidol University's College of Music, and is also a columnist for several magazines, including *Decoration Guide*, *Postcard*, and *Dara Nangbaep*. He contributes and edits his own website, www.niwatkongpien.com, which is an e-magazine that focuses on art criticism, culture, and environmental issues. He is also the manager of the Thai Hornbill Research Foundation, a member of the Cultural Reform Committee, and a consultant for the Thai Film Archive Committee. Niwat serves as a guest lecturer on aesthetics at several Thai universities. He graduated from the Pohchang Academy of Art and undertook further studies on Thai traditional fine arts, particularly, painting and architecture.

RONNAPOOM SAMAKKEEKAROM is a full-time researcher at the Center for Health Policy Studies, with primary research interests in the sexualities of men who love men. He previously worked as a program assistant for the Southeast Asian Consortium on Gender, Sexuality, and Health. He has also been involved in training sessions to build awareness on gender, sexuality, and sexual rights among people of diverse sexualities and genders. He received his master's degree from the Health Social Sciences Program, Mahidol University. With P. Boonmomgkon, he co-authored the chapter "Cyberspace, Power Structure, and Gay Sexual Health," in *Queer Bangkok: 21st Century Markets, Media and Rights* (2011).

SULAIPORN CHONWILAI is an activist and independent researcher. She was previously a member of the editorial staff of *Trendyman* magazine, where she worked on feature articles. She has also worked with an NGO advocating for the rights of homosexual people, and is a member of the Thai Women and HIV/AIDS Task Force. Her research interests include sexuality, lesbian issues, and HIV. She received her master's degree in anthropology from Thammasat University. She is author of *Shifting Sex: Identity, Gender, and Sexuality within a Health Perspective*, prepared for the Center for Health Policy Studies, Mahidol University; and co-editor of *HIV, Community Ways, and Muslim Women* (2007).

TIMO OJANEN was born and raised in Helsinki, Finland. In 2001 he was awarded a B.S. in Psychology with Honors from the University of East London, United Kingdom. After working in two schools in Finland, he moved to Bangkok in 2005, where he studied Thai language and culture at Srinakharinwirot University, and received a master's degree in counseling psychology from Assumption University. He has been active within local sexual/gender minority organizations throughout his time in Thailand, especially the Rainbow Sky Association of Thailand and the Thai Rainbow Archives Project. His current passions include improving the quality of Thai counseling services for sexual/gender minority groups.

INDEX